Mum's NOT having chemo

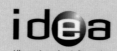

Laura Bond

Mum's NOT having chemo

Cutting-edge therapies, real-life stories –a road-map to healing from cancer

piatkus

This book is dedicated to mum, thank you for your endless patience, limitless love, your wise and wacky spirit and your generous heart. You have made my life a delight and I am very lucky to be your daughter.

PIATKUS

First published in Great Britain in 2013 by Piatkus

A CIP catalogue record for this book
is available from the British Library.

ISBN 978-0-7499-5896-1

Typeset in Stone Serif by M Rules
Printed and bound by CPI Group (UK) Ltd, Croydon, CR0 4YY

Papers used by Piatkus are from well-managed forests
and other responsible sources.

MIX
Paper from
responsible sources
FSC® C104740

Piatkus
An imprint of
Little, Brown Book Group
100 Victoria Embankment
London EC4Y 0DY

An Hachette UK Company
www.hachette.co.uk

www.piatkus.co.uk

The author and publisher have made every effort to ensure the completeness and accuracy of information contained in this book; however, they assume no responsibilities for unwitting errors, omissions or inaccuracies.

This book is for educational purposes only. It is not intended as a substitute for the diagnosis, treatment, or advice from your qualified practitioner. The facts presented in the following pages are offered as information only, not medical advice. If you have cancer, or if you are concerned about cancer, you should seek professional advice.

The author assumes no responsibility for inaccuracies in the source materials, nor in how this material is used. This is not intended to be a comprehensive book, thus it does not claim to contain information on all the possible tests or treatments that could be used for or in relation to cancer.

More information becomes available almost daily and much more may be available by the time you are reading this. To stay in the loop, see the author's website www.mumsnothavingchemo.com.

Contents

Acknowledgements

I'd like to thank both my parents for their unrelenting love and support. Dad for being the voice of reason in a crisis, for encouraging me to follow my dreams and for always being there for me, no matter where I am in the world. Mum for instilling in me a love of healthy food, a passion for writing and a trust in my own intuition.

Thanks also to my siblings for keeping my feet on the ground – Jeremy, Banjo and Emerald. Particular thanks go to Emerald, my little sister, who has painstakingly read every page – and every reference – in this book, giving me honest feedback and spot-on advice. And thanks also to my boyfriend, James, for putting up with endless talk of coffee enemas and for cooking me curry while I worked.

I am also indebted to a legion of courageous doctors and healers who have shared their knowledge so generously. A special mention goes to Dr Garry Gordon, Dr Mark Sircus and Dr Nicholas Gonzalez – their level of support was awesome and unexpected.

Bryan Hubbard and Lynne McTaggart – thank you for the vision you have given to the world, for taking the time to speak with me and for your exhaustive research. I would also like to thank my good friend Jacqui Marson, for her enthusiastic belief in me – and for helping make this book happen.

The support from my team at Piatkus has been tremendous – thank you Anne Lawrance for taking a chance on me and for taking this book into the world. To Anne Newman and Jillian Stewart for whipping my corpulent copy into shape and never once making me feel guilty about it.

For all the supporters of my blog, 'Mum's Not Having Chemo' – without your enthusiasm and feedback this book would not have happened. A special thanks goes to Nicola Corcoran, Patrizia Sergeant and Vincent Crewe, who have rallied behind the book from its inception and responded, without hesitation, to my constant questions.

Foreword by Gemma Bond

Do you see the world through the eyes of a weary traveller or through those of a wonderstruck child? Is your heart full of courage or hopelessness? Gratitude or fear? Hope or despair?

Prior to being ill with cancer, I rarely took the time to question the internal rumblings of dissatisfaction that had been brewing inside me. When my four children started, in turn, to leave home, my sense of purpose left with them, and I didn't consciously register just what a hit my health was taking as a result. It was time for me to rediscover my passion for life, yet I was doggedly resisting the call for change. Cancer turned out to be the catalyst I needed, and my daughter's weekly blog motivated me to stay on the path to wellness and relate to the world in a new, more positive way.

Laura started writing the blog 'Mum's Not Having Chemo' as a way of explaining my decision to say 'No' to mainstream medicine and 'Yes' to ozone therapy, energy healing and more. We both had a burning desire to share some of the information we'd discovered: how these treatments work, which work best – for me, at least – and how they can be used alongside conventional medicine. Although I have always been a fiercely private person, being faced with a life-threatening illness – ovarian and uterine cancer – quickly put paid to my inhibitions and I found I was happy to share details about my morning coffee enemas, regular vitamin injections and reluctant visits to therapy sessions, if it meant even just one person benefited.

To my amazement, the blog touched many. Messages from people all over the world came streaming in like sunlight, filling my daughter and me with hope and joy and transforming my view of the disease. Rather than seeing cancer as a private 'enemy', I came to see it as more of a communal project through which both my readers and I could grow and learn. Each week my daughter would cover a new treatment or topic in the blog, often calling on well-known and respected experts for their advice. The benefits of this were twofold: not only did I have a weekly reminder of the value of the therapies I was already using, but I was also encouraged to look more deeply at treatments I might otherwise have overlooked. As we've passed on information, readers have opened up and shared their own experiences. Some of their stories have been heartbreaking, but many have been immensely uplifting.

Cancer is not a one-size-fits-all ordeal: what works for one person will not necessarily work for the next. But having read dozens of books on the subject, spent hundreds of hours on the internet and having spoken with countless other survivors, I've discovered that overcoming cancer almost always requires a multi-pronged approach. As renowned naturopath and clinical nutritionist David J. Getoff says: 'When a house is falling apart from the inside, a few new doors and windows will not prevent it from tumbling down.'

For me, my illness signalled the need for a major overhaul on a physical, emotional and spiritual level. Prior to getting cancer, I rarely gave myself permission to pause. I was always postponing leisure time in favour of 'one more' task. I would tell myself, 'If I can just get dinner ready/put one more load of washing on/call in on elderly parents/reply to that email ... then I can relax,' but that time almost never came.

Now, I stop myself when I start hearing that internal dialogue and make time to do what I love, whether it's listening to an inspirational speaker on my iPod or walking around the garden barefoot in the mornings, with my dogs and my gardening gloves. I realised following my diagnosis that I had a nature deficit and that spending more time outside not only soothed my soul, but also brought healing vitamin D, fresh oxygen and a dose of magnesium from a dip in the sea. Going to the beach, once fraught with anxiety and preparation, is now a grab-the-keys-and-go affair: no sunscreen, no make-up, no cares. I now wonder how I denied myself such a feel-good experience for so many years, especially since my home in Australia is no more than ten minutes from the beach.

As well as including things that you feel are missing from your life, it is also important to get rid of all those that are bugging you, if you want to be truly healthy. Toxic emotions and people cause harm on a cellular level, leading to chronic low-level stress and preventing much-needed oxygen from getting to our cells. I've discovered that it's not easy to change the way you respond to stress – but I'm finding that the more I see a situation as part of the universe's grand plan, the easier it becomes to let go.

To give you an example, I recently drove for an hour on a very hot Saturday to pick up a new mulcher – not realising the garden centre closed at 12pm. Instead of reacting in a negative way to this as I once would have done, 'post-cancer' Gemma chose to let it go and enjoy the rest of the day. Rather than blaming myself for not checking the opening hours or being annoyed at my boyfriend, I turned to him and said, 'You know what? It's a beautiful day, let's go to the beach.' When we got there the strip was packed and there was not a parking space in sight. We were just about ready to give up and go home when a woman walked past our car jangling her keys and said, 'I'm parked just over here, follow me!' What I'm finding is that, the more I make an effort to let go, the more the universe tends to reach out with a helping hand.

People are always asking me and my daughter whether I'm cured. Many even cast doubts as to whether it's a good idea to publish a book just two years after the initial diagnosis. 'What if it comes back?' is something they don't dare ask, but the question hangs heavy in the air. But in writing this book we felt it was important to show people that we refused to bow to the fear and uncertainty of this disease that so many people cling to. For right from the very moment of diagnosis, it was not the word cancer that made me the most fearful, but the thought of conventional treatment.

I like to think of malignant cells as 'delinquent teenagers', as described by Japanese oncologist Dr Tsuneo Kobayashi (see page 197). The metaphor suggests you need to nurture, nourish and soothe your body, rather than treat it as a war zone. For me, cancer is like any other serious 'life-threatening' disease – like heart disease, high blood pressure or diabetes. People never think to ask those suffering from these conditions, 'Are you cured?' This seems to be a question reserved exclusively for those who've had cancer, while it's assumed that people with other common chronic diseases will be fine so long as they take their medicine, follow the advice of their doctor and 'manage' their condition.

At the time of writing I have just undergone an MRI and blood-marker tests showing that my body is cancer-free. But I'm not getting caught up with being 'cured'. Rather, I like to think I'm managing my condition, and at the moment I seem to be managing it very well . . .

Introduction

The purpose of this book is not to tell you what to do – far from it. It is simply to open your mind to the wide range of healing possibilities, so you can make a decision based on information rather than fear.

When I discovered mum had cancer it was like stepping out of my body and into a nightmare. I recall thrashing my fists against the floor, while my English boyfriend looked on helplessly, not knowing what to say or do. There are no words in that situation that can provide comfort and, for me, the only way to quell the terror was to get online and find a solution.

Google 'cancer treatments' and you will get over 50 million results. For many people, the mass of information is overwhelming, but for mum and me it was thrilling. The more pages I printed out, the more certain I became that mum was going to get better. If the ozone and vitamin C injections didn't work, then we could always try hyperthermia, high-dose turmeric or hemp oil. There's little doubt that my experience as a journalist gave me a head start; the job merged seamlessly with the role of 'cancer secretary': I had access to reliable databases and could call on renowned experts – like Dr Jonathan Wright, Dr Nicholas Gonzalez and Patrick Holford – for advice. But for others, the literature on alternative cancer treatments is like the proverbial rabbit hole.

Since starting the blog 'Mum's Not Having Chemo' I've received hundreds of emails from readers who felt paralysed by conflicting advice, myths and controversy. One subscriber recently posted this comment: 'Thanks for such fantastic, easily readable and accurate info. Wish it had been so easily accessible four years ago when I said no to chemo and radiation! There is just such a minefield out there and it is really tough getting on top of things.'

My hope is that this book, like the blog, will give patients back their voice, their dignity and the confidence to ask questions. We're told that sophisticated treatments are on the horizon, but in fact they are here right now.

In these pages you will hear about a breakthrough heat treatment that demolishes cancer cells by the millions (and leaves healthy cells intact) and an FDA-approved therapy for brain cancer that uses electric fields. You will also learn valuable steps you can take to dramatically decrease your own chance of developing cancer, from daily humming and hydrogen peroxide baths to reducing your toxic load and giving up dairy.

While we all may yearn for the quick fix when disaster strikes, when it comes to cancer there is no magic bullet – and it's unlikely that there ever will be. 'What we need is a medical establishment that diversifies its strategy beyond the exhausted drugs we know don't work,' says author and publisher of the highly acclaimed newsletter *Cancer Defeated!*, Lee Euler. 'In a recent meeting of 100 cancer specialists at the World Oncology Forum in Switzerland, experts at least agreed on one thing: urgent action is needed.'

A baby born today has a one in two chance of developing cancer in his or her lifetime.[1] The 'cut, poison, burn' paradigm may seem like the safest choice, but the truth is that people die as a result of chemotherapy and radiation. The treatments are harsh and the limitations glossed over. In a 2012 survey reported by Reuters at least two-thirds of people with advanced cancer believed the chemotherapy they were receiving might cure them, even though the treatment was only being given to buy some time or make them more comfortable.[2]

Mum has tried many treatments, tools and emotional healing techniques in the two years since her diagnosis. The ones she has found most helpful – like infrared saunas and energy medicine, for example – have made it into this book. Other treatments, like laetrile (apricot kernels), haven't made the cut. But that's not to say that these protocols aren't right for others dealing with the disease. Every cancer is different, every person is different and every treatment plan will be different.

There are many paths to recovery, but through my research and interviews I have found that cancer survivors often responded to their diagnoses in a similar way: they shared a tendency to view their illness not as a death threat, but as a wake-up call, and they showed a willingness to embrace radical, positive change.

While it might be tempting to bury your head in the sand, abdicating responsibility won't help you heal. So rise up, read up and take the reins. The road to health starts with being fully informed.

CHAPTER 1

Accept the Diagnosis
Not the Prognosis

*'Words can become swords and cure
or kill just like a scalpel.'*
Dr Bernie Siegel, author of *Peace, Love and Healing*

March 2011. I've just turned twenty-eight, and I'm back in Australia after five years in London. The conversation, the same one I will have over and over again, goes something like this:

'What are you doing back in Perth?'

'Mum's just had a health scare,' I say, stalling.

Then, putting the person out of their misery, I add: 'We just found out she has ovarian and uterine cancer.'

'Is she having chemo?' they ask, their voice rising in hope.

'No, she's definitely not having chemo.'

Pause.

'Wow, she's brave,' they say. But what they're thinking is: 'She's mad.'

The only thing more shocking than telling someone your mum has cancer is, apparently, revealing that she is not having chemotherapy. Yet ask a group of oncologists (doctors who specialise in the treatment of cancer) what they would do if they were given a diagnosis and their answer might surprise you. In 1986, in a survey conducted by the McGill Cancer Centre in Canada, 64 out of 79 doctors (that's 81 per cent) said in the confidential questionnaire that they would not submit to a common chemotherapy drug, cisplatin, while 58 out of 79 believed that all the therapies offered were not acceptable to them or their family members.[1] Why? Many believed the chemotherapy drugs were ineffective and came with an unacceptable degree of toxicity. A more recent poll by the *Los Angeles Times* came to a similar conclusion. In the survey 75 per cent of oncologists reported that chemotherapy and radiation were unacceptable as treatments for themselves or their families.[2]

This lack of faith in oncological drugs is mirrored elsewhere: Phillip Day, a UK-based health researcher and author of *Cancer: Why We're Still Dying to Know the Truth*, regularly talks with oncologists around the world and most of them admit they would not take their own treatment. 'They're quite forthright about that,' says Day.

At the time of writing, I know of two Australian oncologists with prostate cancer, both of whom are being treated exclusively by a holistic doctor. Can you imagine if their patients knew? How can doctors recommend a therapy they themselves would refuse? The answer is simple. By suggesting patients go outside the box and try alternative cancer treatments, oncologists risk losing their medical licences and livelihoods. 'In Australia and the United States today, doctors can be struck off and sent to jail for "harming their patients' right to life" in using nutrition and lifestyle changes instead of chemotherapy to treat cancer,' says Day. But as a cancer patient you've got a lot to lose too. Your life is at stake.

Going Her Own Way

When mum was first diagnosed, she figured there must have been a mistake. We all did. It just didn't seem possible that someone who had spent decades eating healthy food, practising yoga and riding the zeitgeist of 'crazy' alternative therapies – chakra balancing, kinesiology, cranio-sacral therapy – could get cancer.

It didn't help that her outward symptoms were ruthlessly subtle – ovarian cancer is not called the 'silent killer' for nothing. Mum had been experiencing a faint but persistent drawing pain in her lower abdomen, her periods would stop and start again and she was feeling bloated. She saw her GP and asked to have the CA 125 blood test and a trans-vaginal ultrasound. She'd read years before that these two tests provide the best indication of ovarian cancer. Indeed, in an ongoing study of 200,000 women, British doctors found that using the tests in tandem detected 90 per cent of ovarian cancer cases.[3]

But even after these two tests came back positive mum was convinced the tumour, or whatever the dark mass was that the ultrasound had revealed, wasn't really anything to worry about. That is until the night following her hysterectomy. The surgeon, who'd spent the evening poring over mum's pathology report, delivered the diagnosis: that she had ovarian cancer and it was in her uterus too. Mum broke down in tears.

Mum's Diagnosis: the Details

According to the pathology report mum had cancer in one ovary that had spread to her uterus. The pathologist was not able to confirm whether the cancer was stage 1 or stage 3, as it depended on whether both tumours were primary and synchronous (had developed at the same

▶

time) or whether the ovarian cancer had metastasised to the uterus. The cancer also showed up in mum's pelvic wash (where the pelvic cavity is 'washed' to check for cancer cells that have moved beyond the cancer point of origin), but not in her lymph nodes.

When mum underwent the full hysterectomy a week after the ominous ultrasound, she insisted on having key-hole surgery, as she understood this would minimise the risk of the cancer spreading. Immediately following the surgery, mum began a course of intravenous vitamin C, which, according to experts, can 'mop up' any rogue cancer cells remaining after an operation (see Chapter 4).

When mum was first diagnosed in March 2011, her CA 125 (a protein found at elevated levels in those who have ovarian cancer – see page 194) was 224. The normal range is 0–21. Six months later her CA 125 result was 8, and two years later an MRI confirmed no cancer in mum's body. Her CA 125 remains normal.

'It's a very aggressive form of cancer, and I'd really urge you to have chemo,' said the surgeon. Through her tears mum managed to blurt out, 'I'm not having chemo.' Now it's one thing to tell yourself you'll never have chemotherapy, but it's quite another matter, when your life is hanging in the balance and you're hooked to a morphine drip, to tell a leading gynaecological oncologist that you won't be taking his advice.

Mum spent those first two weeks agonising over whether she was being stupidly self-righteous. It didn't help that almost everyone – best friends, Chinese and Western doctors alike – were all shaking their heads in despair. But us kids? We supported mum from the start. Having grown up in a house where vitamins and ouija breathing were used to treat everything from sore throats to broken hearts – and where it was normal to find mum upside down in a headstand machine or supervising the dog's acupuncture – we knew that the natural way was the only way for mum.

After years of eye rolling and scepticism, my brothers, sister and I had come to trust in mum's unconventional advice. We'd reluctantly dissolved homeopathic tablets under our tongues, and watched as mosquito bites vanished; rubbed Swedish bitters on our foreheads, too hung over to argue, and felt migraines lift; we'd begrudgingly booked in for 'vitamin cocktails' to ward off the flu while all around us fell ill ... We believed alternative medicine could work.

The Truth about Your Choices

Mum's knowledge of natural medicine provided a glimmer of hope in those dark hours in hospital. She knew of doctors defeating cancer with vitamin C and hydrogen peroxide, and had heard of end-stage cancer patients who'd travelled to alternative clinics in Mexico and Germany and returned tumour-free. She'd never expected, not in her wildest nightmares, to need the information, but in those grim days following her diagnosis, she was glad she had it. There were choices.

Sadly, for most cancer patients there are only three options: cut, poison or burn: statistics reveal 67 per cent of cancer patients submit to surgery, 80 per cent receive chemotherapy and 60 per cent have radiation.[4] And yet, with the exception of Hodgkin's disease, acute lymphocytic leukaemia and testicular cancer, as well as a few rare cancers,[5] chemotherapy makes little difference to long-term survival (i.e. at least five years beyond diagnosis of the primary disease). One major study, published in the *Scientific American* in 1985, found that chemotherapy was 'somewhat effective' in only 2–3 per cent of cancer patients.[6]

But worse than that, chemotherapy can kill. A 2008 British study conducted by the National Confidential Enquiry into Patient Outcomes and Deaths found that chemotherapy actually contributes to a quarter of cancer deaths.[7] In addition, the late Dr Hardin B. Jones, one of the world's top statisticians, led a twenty-five-year study which found that 'untreated cancer victims live up to four times longer than treated individuals'.[8]

Far from being a fringe conspiracy, the ineffectiveness of chemotherapy is acknowledged by some of today's most popular and brilliant minds. In the best-selling book *SuperFreakonomics* Steven D. Levitt and Stephen J. Dubner mention that a typical chemotherapy regime for non-small-cell lung cancer costs more than $40,000, but helps extend a patient's life by an average of just two months. They write: '... it is easy to envision a point in the future, perhaps fifty years from now, when we collectively look back at the early twenty-first century's cutting-edge cancer treatments and say: We were giving our patients *what*?'[9]

Even those at the heart of conventional medicine acknowledge the limitations of cancer drugs. In April 2012 Dr Otis Brawley, Chief Medical and Scientific Officer of the American Cancer Society (ACS), criticised mainstream cancer treatments. In a speech to health journalists he admitted that doctors frequently lie about the success rates of both screenings and treatments – including PSA exams for prostate cancer, bone marrow transplants and chemotherapy[10] – calling the current system 'a subtle form of corruption'.

So where were the front-page headlines? Sadly, the other side of the story rarely makes the news. Instead, we are told that a cure for cancer is 'just around the corner' and that survival rates are improving. In November 2011 Macmillan Cancer Support released a paper stating that: 'Overall median survival time for all cancer types forty years ago was just one year, now it is predicted to be nearly six years.'[11] So should we applaud the apparent progress, or should we, like Phillip Day, take the statistics with a pinch of salt? 'Torture the data long enough and eventually it will confess to anything,' quips Day.

Doctored Figures

Certain factors give official figures a brighter sheen: we are now catching cancer at an earlier stage, which means patients are not necessarily living longer after they get cancer, rather, they're living longer *after they are diagnosed* with the disease; non-invasive cancers like ductal carcinoma in situ (DCIS) – also known as 'zero-grade cancer'[12] – are included in statistics; and the word 'survive' has been redefined to mean only five years.

'My aunt – who had all the chemo offered – is forever immortalised as a breast cancer "survivor",' says Day. 'She survived the five years, but died six months after that. So she's "cured" and dead.'

Twenty-five years ago Day embarked upon a worldwide quest to find the 'answer' to cancer. The result? He discovered the clinics getting the best results were focusing on nutrition, stress management and lifestyle changes. 'They weren't doing chemotherapy and radiation at all. That surprised me,' says Day.

'Chemo Saved My Life'

Of course, it goes without saying that conventional treatment works for some people. We all have friends or loved ones and know of celebrities who've chosen the conventional route and are doing well. When Olivia Newton-John was diagnosed with breast cancer she opted for surgery and eight months of chemotherapy. Today, more than twenty years later, she is still gracing magazine covers having not only defied her diagnosis but also, it would seem, the ravages of ageing.

But chemotherapy is rarely the whole story: 'The

chemotherapy might have shrunk the tumour to the point where the patient is sent home, but what's never recorded is whether the patient, having had a major lifestyle wake-up call, improves their diet, starts exercising and looks after themselves better,' Phillip Day surmises.

The Tumour is Not the Problem

If a doctor says to you, 'This drug has a 90 per cent response rate,' you'd feel pretty reassured, right? Why look at other options with those encouraging odds? But it pays to check you're on the same page as your oncologist. When they tell you a chemotherapy drug has a 90 per cent response rate they're simply talking about the likelihood that the tumour will decrease in size. What happens to you? That's another matter entirely.

Renowned medical researcher Ralph W. Moss discovered that chemotherapy can lead to meaningful life extension in about ten different forms of cancer. However, most of these cancers are rare. For the common solid tumours (like breast, ovarian and prostate cancers – those responsible for 90 per cent of all cancer deaths) chemotherapy is not effective.[13] Your tumour might respond, but you might die.

'The conventional people drive me nuts,' says leading cancer specialist Dr Nicholas Gonzalez. 'They approach cancer like a nuclear war, as if you've got to "nuke every single cell", and they end up killing the patient as well.' Dr Gonzalez has patients who have been with him for fifteen years who still have tumours. 'They [the tumours] are quiet; they could be dead, but they're not bothering anybody, as long as the patient takes their enzymes, they're fine.' (See Chapter 4 for more on enzymes.)

▶

The bottom line? Tumour-size reduction should not be the main priority: 'The focus must switch to survival and quality of life. Focusing on making a tumour shrink with chemo/radiation is a fool's game,' says Dr Garry Gordon, co-founder of the American College for Advancement in Medicine (ACAM).

One of my blog readers, Lee Gefen, a thirty-four-year-old woman from Australia, has chosen to view her (inoperable) brain tumour as a need for change: 'I no longer feel like the tumour is threatening me, or invading me or that I have to fight it. I am learning to live with it in peace, while doing everything I can to treat what caused it in the first place.' (See Chapter 12 for more inspiring stories.)

When faced with cancer, most patients want to pull out all the stops, and increasingly that means stopping by the reiki healer or Chinese doctor and taking potent supplements. A recent survey at MD Anderson Cancer Center, found an astounding 83 per cent of patients were using alternative medicine alongside conventional treatments.[14] Yet these added extras are never considered in cancer statistics. Instead, 'progress' is pinned exclusively on medical advancements and not to patient initiative.

For Newton-John, meditation, homeopathy, acupuncture and relaxation techniques were just some of the healing therapies she turned to following conventional treatment.[15] She also reportedly takes digestive enzymes and vitamin D daily (see Chapter 4) and is passionate about eating healthy, organic food. While Newton-John managed to bounce back from chemotherapy, many more don't. According to Ciaran Devane, CEO of Macmillan Cancer Support: 'Cancer treatment is the toughest fight many people will face and patients are often left with long-term health and emotional problems long after their treatment has ended.'

Leukaemia, heart failure and infertility are just some of the listed side effects of doxorubicin, a common chemotherapy drug, while 5 FU, another one, is so toxic some doctors refer to it as 'Five Feet Under'.[16] While we constantly read about 'new breakthrough treatments', the reality is that many patients are offered drugs that are decades old. One of my blog readers from the UK, Jayne Brown, was shocked to discover that the same chemotherapy drug used unsuccessfully on her late partner in 1993 was given to her friend in 2007. 'I am incredulous that with twelve additional years of research, the chemo cocktail given to my partner is still part of mainstream medicine,' says Brown.

It's worth bearing in mind that up to three-quarters of all published research on pharmaceutical drugs in the medical literature is now believed to be ghost-written by public relations firms, hired by drug companies.[17] The fact that cancer is profitable to many – more than $40 billion is spent worldwide each year on cancer drugs[18] – is a truth that cannot be ignored. 'Chemotherapy is certainly good for the balance sheets of pharmaceutical companies. It builds careers. It may even offer patients and their families hope in hopeless times. But it is not an effective weapon against the vast majority of solid carcinomas in adults,' according to acclaimed medical journalist Ralph Moss.[19]

But most of us don't ask questions: 'Patients are often vulnerable, frightened and don't fully understand their disease,' says Kathryn Alexander, naturopath, detoxification expert and author of *Dietary Healing: The Complete Detox Program*. 'When I ask patients why they have chosen certain treatments they will often say, "The doctor seemed so nice". While it is obviously better to have a kind specialist than one who is abrupt and rude, being nice does not qualify as a treatment, and the advice given needs to be properly evaluated.'

Tunnel vision can take over when you receive a diagnosis. Thoughts turn to friends or loved ones who lost the battle and hopelessness sets in like rising damp; any reservations about conventional treatment vanish and fear takes hold. Suddenly, any option sounds like a good one, even if it comes with death as a 'side effect'. Radiation? Bring it on. Surgery? Sign me up. Cancer-causing chemicals? You bet.

'Every day we get dozens of calls from people all over the world,' says New York-based physician Dr Nicholas Gonzalez. 'These people did all the "right" things – the surgery, the chemo – now the cancer is in their brain and their lungs and their liver. They're scared and they've started to look into alternatives.'

Why Cancer Comes Back

A 2012 study shows that chemotherapy damages healthy cells, causing them to secrete a protein that accelerates the growth of cancer tumours.[20] This protein, called 'WNT16B' causes them to 'grow, invade, and importantly, resist subsequent therapy', according to Peter Nelson of the Fred Hutchinson Cancer Research Center in Seattle. Nelson is co-author of the study that observed this phenomenon, published in Nature Medicine.[21]

Radiotherapy has long been linked to secondary cancers. It's now well documented that a woman whose breast is irradiated is more likely to develop lung cancer.[22] If that wasn't bad enough, radiotherapy can ultimately generate a more aggressive type of cancer. 'Radiotherapy has been shown to increase the survival and self-renewing capacity of breast cancer cells by up to thirty-fold,' says Sayer Ji, founder and director of GreenMedInfo.com and co-author of the book The Cancer Killers: The Cause Is The Cure. 'This means that while radiation treatment may initially regress a tumour's volume/mass, it may actually be

▶

selecting out the more radiation-resistant and aggressive subpopulation of tumour cells which ultimately lead to higher malignancy.'[23]

The latest research is now suggesting that chemotherapy and radiation are not capable of treating the slow-growing cancer 'stem cells' (the mostly deadly type of cell within a tumour). In fact, chemotherapy and radiation may well lead to a rise in their ranks.[24] Thankfully, there are promising natural treatments – like Haelan (see Chapter 8) – which *are* capable of demolishing cancer stem cells, according to preliminary research.

Embracing Health vs Fighting Disease

We've collectively bought into the idea that harm caused by the healer is an inevitable part of the 'battle' against cancer. But it doesn't have to be this way. For the last twenty-five years, Dr Gonzalez has been treating cancer patients with individualised diets, enzymes and coffee enemas – with phenomenal success.

'I have patients now in their mid-nineties that have been with me for twenty years,' says Dr Gonzalez. 'I have a woman with pancreatic cancer who lives in Texas. I haven't seen her in about eight years, but she always sends me a Christmas card.'

Why We Get Cancer: Old Thinking vs New Thinking

Old thinking: genetic weakness New thinking: epigenetic changes

▶

Old thinking: sunbaking **New thinking**: not enough vitamin D

Old thinking: missing mammograms **New thinking**: having mammograms

Old thinking: high-fat diet **New thinking**: highly processed diet

Old thinking: stress doesn't matter **New thinking**: stress is a root cause

Old thinking: the cure is drugs **New thinking**: the cure is the immune system

---

When mum first decided to stray from the conventional path, she assumed it would be a lonely journey. How wrong she was! We quickly discovered the alternative cancer community is a thriving population, which is driving demand for holistic practitioners worldwide. Indeed, according to research published in *Australian Family Physician*, patients in Australia now visit alternative practitioners almost as frequently as they do their GP. Professor Ian Brighthope, a leading medical doctor and surgeon, has witnessed a dramatic change in public opinion in the last thirty-five years: 'It has been interesting to see how something like high-dose vitamin C – once regarded as absolute quackery – has become mainstream,' he says.

Around the world, the natural health movement is rapidly gaining momentum. Britons now spend £450 million a year on complementary and alternative medicine, and in America sales of organic food and beverages have grown from $1 billion in 1990 to $26.7 billion in 2010.[25] People are hungry for real, unprocessed food along with unadulterated information about their health-care options. Thankfully, reliable research is now available through leading health news hubs like Natural News.com and Mercola.com. Boasting millions of readers, these websites are able to disseminate leading health news at breakneck speed. With more and more information available, patients are now arriving at appointments with printouts and a list of questions to ask, rather than simply an array of symptoms to treat.

Making important medical decisions can be exceptionally stressful and at times incredibly lonely, but this book will help you navigate the darkness. You will find details of cutting-edge alternative treatments – like hyperthermia and ozone therapy (see Chapters 7 and 9) – which have reversed countless cases of 'terminal' cancer. I will also touch on the exciting field of molecular oncology and mention a groundbreaking technique which allows doctors to identify cancer cells years before normal marker tests (see Chapter 10). At the back of the book you will find a helpful Resources section with lots of information on the tests, treatments, clinics and specialists mentioned in the text.

You may be surprised to learn that when a person is diagnosed with cancer they have usually been living with the disease for an average of seven years. This certainly undermines the common belief that the tumour is a ticking time bomb requiring *immediate* removal. 'It's a very slow-growing disease, and patients should be patient,' cautions American physician and nutrition expert Dr John A. McDougall.

Dr Patrick Kingsley, British cancer expert and author of *The New Medicine,* offers similar advice: 'If you've just been given a diagnosis of cancer, sit back and think about what you want to do. It won't make the slightest bit of difference if you don't do anything for the first week or two, but it gives you a chance to think whether you want to follow the advice your doctor is giving you, get a second opinion or follow your own way of doing things.'

In these pages you will hear from an Australian woman who rid herself of a tumour using only a black salve (see page 247), a German man who treated his pancreatic cancer with homeopathy (see page 249) and an English woman who chose apricot kernels over chemotherapy (see page 256). I've had the privilege of speaking to many cancer patients who've defied a death sentence and I now firmly believe that where there is hope, there is healing. Sadly, some physicians, wary of giving 'false hope', take away this essential ingredient for recovery. Dr James Forsythe isn't one of them. In *Take Control of Your Cancer* he writes, 'I always try to err on the side of optimism with patients. I've had patients come to me saying their doctors had told them not to start a new novel or start watching a new soap opera because they wouldn't be alive long enough to see the ending.'

Prognoses are based on statistics, but there are always exceptions. 'Terminal' cancer patients – with metastases to the bones, lungs and liver – have been known to fully recover, pancreatic tumours have vanished and those who've been sent home to die have gone on to live.

So what should you do if a physician tells you, 'There's nothing more we can do'? Dr Keith Scott-Mumby, author of *Cancer Research Secrets,* suggests the following: 'If a doctor ever says such words to you, translate them as follows: "I don't know what I'm talking about and I don't know what I'm doing. I suggest you find a natural healer and follow a spiritual and lifestyle path to a cure."'

●

CHAPTER 2

The Cancer Personality

*'I can't express anger. I internalise it
and grow a tumour instead.'*
Woody Allen, *Manhattan*

Are you eager to please, easily worried and feel like your life lacks meaning? Do you find it difficult to forgive, ask for favours and say 'No'? All of us struggle with these things from time to time. But if you habitually find yourself putting others first and burying your real feelings, you might be increasing your odds of getting cancer.

Dr Rashid A. Buttar, renowned physician, detox expert and author of *The 9 Steps to Keep the Doctor Away*, jokes that his ex-wife will never get breast cancer. Why? According to him, she simply doesn't fit the personality profile. After treating hundreds of breast cancer patients, Buttar discovered they shared certain traits: 'Nearly all the women were constantly giving of themselves and were always worried about something. The stress never ended. If one thing they had worried about was resolved, they found three new things to replace it. I also noted that they never, ever took any time off for themselves.'

For award-winning cancer counsellor Dr Susan Silberstein, the cancer/stress connection is undeniable: 'We ask patients, "Why do you think you got sick?" Ninety-five per cent of them say they knew exactly where the disease came from: stress.'[1]

Ancient wisdom and common sense tell us that feelings of hopelessness, frustration and anxiety can destroy our immune systems and wreak havoc on our health. When tension headaches take hold or when our skin suddenly breaks out we'll shrug our shoulders and admit we're 'under a lot of pressure' or 'stressed to the max', but now science is giving credence to this intuitive connection: research from Stanford University Medical School reveals that 95 per cent of all illness is stress-related.[2] And yet, when it comes to cancer, we can't shake the belief that stress is irrelevant and that smoking, bad genes and bad luck are the best predictors of the disease. Nothing could be further from the truth: 'The genes don't make the decision,' says Dr Bernie Siegel, cancer surgeon and best-selling author. 'They're stimulated by the internal chemistry, which is called epigenetics.'

The epigenome is located on top of the genome (hence the prefix 'epi', meaning above). We now know that environmental factors like diet and stress can switch genes on and off. 'We can't change our genes, but we can change their function and expression,' writes Dr Mark Hyman in his book *The Blood Sugar Solution*. 'The collective experience of our lives – our intrauterine environment, diet, toxins, microbes, allergens, stresses, social connections, thoughts and beliefs – controls which genes are turned on and off.' In a 2001 survey of nearly 400 Canadian breast cancer patients, 42 per cent cited stress as one of the main causes of their disease, considerably more than blamed either genetic or environmental causes.[3]

Genes or Lifestyle?

Genes do not control your destiny – that's the take-home message from the exciting field of epigenetics: 'The vast majority of diseases we suffer from – diabetes, obesity,

▶

heart disease, cancer – are multifactorial lifestyle diseases,' says integrative health specialist Chris Kresser. 'Genetics may determine our predisposition to these conditions, but those genes must be activated (or silenced) by environmental triggers such as diet and stress in order to cause disease.'

From the moment we enter the womb to the last seconds of life, our genes are susceptible to change. The new science of foetal origins reveals that what a mother eats during pregnancy can affect everything from a child's IQ and temperament to their bone structure and hair colour. But what goes on in a mother's mind also has an impact. Depression, anxiety, grief and trauma all have the potential to leave a genetic imprint on the baby. One recent study suggested that pregnant women who developed post-traumatic stress disorder (PTSD) following 9/11 had children who were more likely to develop PTSD following a traumatic event themselves.[4]

According to Dr Leonard Coldwell, who has reached an audience of over 57 million with his books and seminars and is considered a leading authority on stress-related illness, gestational stress can be carcinogenic. Coldwell, who boasts a 92.3 per cent success rate for treating cancer patients, explains: 'If the mother is very stressed during pregnancy the body is deprived of oxygen and therefore the foetus is deprived of oxygen.' And we now know that one of the main causes of cancer is lack of oxygen (see Chapter 9). One long-term Danish study raises further questions about the idea that genes are the most important factor. When researchers looked at the medical history of almost 1000 adopted children born between 1924 and

▶

1926 they discovered that children were more likely to die prematurely of cancer (before the age of fifty) if their adopted parents died prematurely of the disease. However, the researchers found no such correlation with their biological parents.[5]

Today, the lifetime risk of breast cancer among females with the BRCA1 and BRCA2 gene is 82 per cent. But the statistics haven't always been so dire. 'Before 1940, that same BRCA2 gene only expressed in about 24 per cent of cases,'[6] says Dr Alexander Mostovoy, Toronto-based homeopathic physician and thermographer. 'So what's changed in the last fifty years? Genetically humans don't change ... the only thing that's changing is our environment.'

Dr Thomas Lodi, an integrative oncologist from Arizona, has a similar view: 'What "runs" in families are eating habits and lifestyles – like eating pasta and white bread. One hundred years ago, 0.5 per cent of Americans got cancer. Almost 50 per cent of Americans alive today will get cancer in their lifetimes. Where is the genetics in that?' he says.

Junk food and junk thoughts, coupled with increased pollution and radiation, all have a hand in disease. Indeed, one recent study found that women exposed to high levels of radiation (to treat Hodgkin's lymphoma) were more likely to develop breast cancer than those who carried the BRCA1 mutation.[7]

'By blaming genes for disease, doctors disempower patients and convince them that they have no control over their own health,' says Dr Zenon Gruba, a qualified physician who has been studying natural medicine for the last forty years. 'The truth is that you can be free of cancer

▶

regardless of your genetic code, because it is the expression of those genes that matters.'

Focusing on what's right, rather than what's wrong, might be the key to better health: 'Diet, a strong social network, purposeful work, mental stimulation and an environment free of toxins might be far more important than the genes you're born with,'[8] summarises best-selling author, Lynne McTaggart.

The fact that genes do not control your destiny might explain why one twin develops breast cancer while the other remains healthy. 'If you have twin sisters and one is a submissive young lady, who tries to please her parents and never expresses anger, but her sister is a little devil and doesn't care what anyone thinks, who's more likely to get cancer? The answer is, the good girl,' says Dr Bernie Siegel, who has devoted his life to understanding the emotional aspects of cancer.

There is now a slew of journals dedicated to the emerging fields of psycho-oncology and psychoneuroimmunology (PNI) and pioneering researchers like Dr Bruce Lipton, David Hamilton and Dr Joan Borysenko are using science to prove the mind–body connection. 'People never thought that stress could have a direct effect on cancer,' says Dr Joan Borysenko, a Harvard-trained medical scientist, psychologist and author of *Fried: Why You Burn Out and How to Revive*. 'But it turns out that when you're stressed, the enzymes that repair breaks in DNA are affected, so you can't repair damaged DNA as easily.'

Adrenaline – the 'fight-or-flight' hormone – can even make cancer resistant to treatment, according to one recent study. In a paper published in the journal *Cancer Genetics and Cytogenetics* in April 2009,[9] researchers from a university in China showed that adrenaline, secreted at times of stress, induced multi-drug resistance in colon cancer cells. The stress hormone epinephrine has also been shown to alter prostate and breast cancer cells in ways that makes them resistant to cell death, according to a study published in the *Journal of Biological Chemistry* in 2007.[10]

'But how do I avoid stress?' I hear you shout, exasperated. 'I have three kids, a demanding job, parents to look after: life is stressful.' While it's true that our lives are becoming increasingly stretched and cortisol levels are collectively skyrocketing, it is possible to make choices – big and small – to reshape our psychological landscape and daily reality. Dr Leonard Coldwell believes *emotional* stress is the root cause of cancer in 86 per cent of all cases. 'When I say mental and emotional stress I mean living with constant worries, doubts and fears, making compromises against yourself, staying in a relationship that you know is wrong, going to a job that you know is going to kill you.'

Most deadly heart attacks happen Monday morning between 8 and 9am, according to research: 'They happen when people are getting ready to go to a job they cannot handle any more: they would rather die, literally, than go to that job one more time,' says Coldwell. How often have you heard someone say, 'This job/marriage is killing me?' We see it as a throwaway line, but according to experts it's our subconscious speaking – and we should listen up.

When Dr Bernie Siegel asks patients to describe their experience of cancer, the words they use can be telling: 'For some it might be "failure", "roadblock", "draining". For others it might be "wake-up call", "blessing", "new beginning",' he says. 'So I ask the people on the negative side: "What's causing you pressure?" and they'll say, "Pressure? Oh, my marriage" or "I've felt like a failure since childhood – my parents committed suicide." When they understand the meaning behind the words it helps them heal their life – and sometimes their illness too ... One patient, close to death, described her disease as "an obstruction". I suggested that she needed to deal with all the obstructions in her life,' says Siegel. Five days later the woman left hospital. Nine months later she was still alive. 'Although I've lost track of her since, I feel sure that she did indeed deal with the obstructions in her life.'

To onlookers, mum's life appeared problem-free: she had four healthy children, a good relationship and enough money. And yet she came to realise that from an early age, anxiety and worry could often overwhelm her. Understanding that these emotional factors may have contributed to her cancer was hugely empowering for mum. It gave her something to work on. Since she already led a healthy lifestyle – eating organic, exercising, avoiding alcohol – mum initially felt disillusioned when she developed cancer. 'What more can I do?' she asked. But when she realised that stress and negative rumination were as carcinogenic as any MSG-laden takeaway, she went about transforming her mindset.

So is there really such a thing as the cancer-prone personality? Psychologist Lydia Temoshok identified thirteen 'non-verbal characteristics' that distinguish the 'Type C' personality; according to her studies, these behavioural patterns are linked with thicker, more invasive tumours than those in non-Type C patients.[11] Dr Lawrence LeShan, regarded as the pioneer of psychological support for cancer, frequently predicts the presence of cancer by personality profile alone.

Not every cancer patient will relate to the characteristics described in this chapter, and environmental toxins, junk food and damaged genes do also have a role to play. But for those who *do* identify with the Type C personality profile, take heart. These words are not here to blame (the last thing you need when you're dealing with something like cancer), but rather to inspire change. As renowned speaker and author Dr Christiane Northrup so aptly says: 'We are not so much responsible for our illnesses as responsible *to* them.' Cancer is a multifactorial disease and getting on top of your emotional health is just one more step you can take towards healing.

Defining the Type C Personality

In this chapter we focus on five defining characteristics of the 'Type C personality', while in Chapter 3, we uncover psychological tools other survivors have used to gain a foothold in their recovery. The five characteristics are:

- Always putting others first

- Low self-esteem

- Bottling up emotions

- Living in fear

- Harbouring resentment

Always putting others first: the 'have-to-please' disease?

A tendency to put others first is common among cancer patients, according to numerous experts: 'I find with cancer patients ... they're trying to put all their energy into fixing other people's problems while ignoring their own,' said Ayurvedic practitioner and medical intuitive Andreas Moritz.[12] Moritz was the bestselling author of numerous books, including *The Amazing Liver and Gallbladder Flush* and *Cancer is Not a Disease – It's a Survival Mechanism.*

Lydia Temoshok describes the Type C coping style as 'abrogating one's own needs in favour of those of others, suppressing negative emotions ... ' She goes on to say the Type C personality is 'nice, friendly and helpful to others, and rarely gets into arguments or fights'.

For Dr Alexander Mostovoy, who has been studying the cancer personality for over fifteen years, the classic cancer patient is a 'kind soul ... It's your typical mum. She is always helping everybody else in the family, and she comes last.'

Prior to getting cancer, mum felt as if she was 'just going through the motions'. She had no creative outlet, no career and no recognition for working behind the scenes to ensure everyone else's lives ran smoothly. Having invested three decades in us, her four children – making moussaka, writing school speeches and supporting our dreams – mum was left floundering when we became independent adults and started to leave the nest.

Interestingly, a study from the University of Oregon School of Public Health found that housewives had a 154 per cent higher incidence of cancer than females working outside the home.[13] 'The researchers looked for a carcinogen in the kitchen, but there wasn't any,' says Bernie Siegel. 'The possibility that the housewife's feelings of being trapped might be contributing to the higher rate of cancer was never considered . . .'

Two important messages can be gleaned here: first, that it's vital to have a purpose in life and secondly, that purpose should be more meaningful than simply living a 'role', whether that's a mother or market analyst. For Siegel, a cancer diagnosis is a chance for someone to get in touch with their 'authentic' self and rediscover experiences or activities that encourage them to 'live in the moment'.

So how do you translate that noble intention into tangible change? Mum and I have found kundalini yoga a wonderful way to detach from personal concerns and let go (see Chapter 7, page 142). The practice encourages students to leave their ego off the mat, close their eyes and do fast and repetitive exercises to 'release the spirit within'. Taken to the extreme, dancing can also lead to altered states of consciousness: 'In these trance-like states, people become immersed in the group beat,' says Professor Lawrence Parsons, who has spent years researching the neuroscience and psychology of dance. 'You're breathing fast, you're moving hard, your emotions are alive and the music allows you to focus on a few elemental things – all the other parts of your brain shut down.'

Mum's cancer heralded a new order – one where she learned to say 'No' to a packed schedule and 'Yes' to joy and personal fulfilment: she started studying to become a holistic health counsellor and booked a ticket to Europe for the following year so she had something to look forward to. When doubt and worry took hold, she would try and imagine herself strolling through the streets of Paris with her two daughters. She also refused to get caught up in other people's dramas: 'It's not me, it's not mine, I surrender it to the universe,' became mum's daily affirmation.

Low self-esteem

'I have yet to meet a cancer patient who does not feel burdened by low self-esteem, a sense of not being "good enough",' said Andreas Moritz. 'That comes across in many different ways: people become negative, they might try to constantly please others or they might have a deep sense of insecurity. When you don't feel good about yourself the immune system becomes suppressed.'

Dr Mostovoy has a similar view: 'The "C" type personality often needs acceptance from other people – they might have a sense of being unworthy.' If your head is filled with negative self-talk, a cancer diagnosis might lead to more chastising – such as 'How did I let this happen?' or 'What have I done to deserve this?' If you can relate to this mindset, you might want to consider seeking professional support. Many patients turn to psychotherapy as a way of coping with a cancer diagnosis, but few realise the sessions might do more than provide an emotional crutch. Stanford psychiatrist Dr David Spiegel found that women with advanced breast cancer lived twice as long if they had weekly psychotherapy support.[14] And Dr Bernie Siegel knows the mind matters: 'I found that psychiatrists were the ones who wrote books about helping people heal,' he says. 'The therapy ended up prolonging their life and even curing them in some cases.' (See Chapter 3 for more tools.)

For some, low self-esteem is deeply rooted. A few years ago researchers asked a group of Harvard students one simple question: did your parents love you? Ninety-eight per cent of those who answered 'No' suffered a major illness by the time they were middle-aged, as opposed to just 25 per cent of those who said 'Yes'. 'With most illnesses it's growing up without love,' says Bernie Siegel. 'The insecurity can stem from indifference, rejection or abuse.'

So can you blame your parents for getting sick? Of course you can, but it won't help you heal. Making peace with an emotionally absent or abusive mother, however, just might. 'In my experience clients can get stuck feeling angry and sad about their childhoods – they're waiting for an apology from their parents that may never come,' says counselling psychologist Jacqui Marson. She invites such clients to treat themselves with the care and devotion they bestow on others: 'Do you take the time to walk your dog or cook a beautiful meal for your own kids? If you do, then you know how to show love, and that's how you need to look after yourself.'

Bottling up emotions

Reality TV might lead you to think we're pretty good at expressing our emotions these days. But when it comes to deeply upsetting or traumatic experiences (not just being told by Simon Cowell that we 'haven't got it'), many of us would rather choke back the tears than fully embrace the despair. But suppressing these unpleasant feelings can be dangerous: 'Unresolved issues –

frustration, anger, hurt – burn inside a person and form almost like an abscess,' says Dr Rashid Buttar. 'In my experience every person that suffers from cancer has some issue like that. I didn't believe that fifteen years ago, but I do now.' Recent research lends weight to Dr Buttar's observations. A study published in the *Journal of Personality* shows that women with breast cancer who are able to express their anger, fear, sadness and affection in a group setting live longer than those who suppress these emotions.[15]

Casey Terry, a psychologist and reiki master based in Australia, agrees that blocked energy can turn cancerous: 'Unexpressed emotions, unresolved traumas, will try and find a way out. I do believe that cancers often come from suppressed energy – in one form or another.' According to Dr Bernie Siegel, the bodies of people who live very quiet, controlled lives sometimes rebel against them: 'I suggested to one patient that if he made a little more noise in his life, maybe he wouldn't need something "wild" inside of him.'

Psychologists have long known that resolving emotional issues is often the key to cancer recovery. In *You Can Fight for Your Life: Emotional Factors in the Treatment of Cancer*, Dr Lawrence LeShan writes: 'Many of the patients expressed the idea that for years they had felt there was no way out of the emotional box they found themselves in.' LeShan noticed that the majority of his patients had lost their enthusiasm for life. He subsequently developed a new form of therapy, based on over forty years of clinical research and focused on helping a person rediscover their zest for life and 'find their song'[16] (see Chapter 3).

When faced with life-threatening events many of us believe it's important to 'carry on as normal'. But this idea of 'staying strong' in order to get well made no sense to holistic practitioner Andreas Moritz: 'Do not try to pacify the patient and tell him, "It is all going to be okay" ... Let him have his experience of pain, despair, confusion, loneliness, hopelessness, anger, fear, guilt or shame. If the afflicted person knows that he or she can have all these feelings without having to hide them from you or push them right back inside, cancer can become a very powerful means of self-healing.'

Holding back tears of frustration, hurt or anger can be toxic, according to Moritz, the chemical make-up of tears being influenced by our emotional state: 'The tears of joy have pleasure hormones in them, while the tears of pain contain stress hormones ... So when we release tears of frustration that's a fantastic release of toxins.'

The way we handle grief might also affect our future health. In one recently published study, 50 per cent of breast cancer patients had suffered a major traumatic event – such as bereavement – within the previous five years.[17] In another study breast cancer patients reporting one or more traumatic or stressful events had a median disease-free interval of thirty-one months compared with sixty-two months for patients with no such events. The study, from the University of Rochester, was reported in the *Journal of Psychosomatic Research* in 2007.[18]

Some have witnessed first-hand the carcinogenic effect of grief. At the age of sixty-five Dr Mostovoy's aunt was diagnosed with breast cancer – two years after losing her son to cancer. 'He was the father of three young children and passed away following five rounds of chemotherapy,' says Mostovoy. 'What parent is not going to be affected by losing their one and only child? I'm not saying this is the *only* cause, but is this a coincidence? I don't think so.' At some point, all of us are faced with the unparalleled agony of losing a loved one. But not all of us will go on to develop cancer. So what makes grief carcinogenic? 'How we deal with it determines how it will affect our health,' says Mostovoy. 'When you help someone make peace with what happened, hopefully their system self-corrects and brings them back to health and life.'

Living in fear

'Fear is a big thing,' says Mostovoy. 'Over the years I've seen many people [and] it's not really cancer that kills them; it's fear that kills them. You can see it in their eyes. You can see who's going to survive and whose eyes are so full of fears that … it's going to be an uphill battle.' It's a bold statement, but one that's recently been supported by science. In April 2012 the *New England Journal of Medicine* published a study showing that the anxiety induced by a cancer diagnosis can be as deadly as the cancer itself. The Swedish research analysed more than 500,000 people who were diagnosed with cancer between 1991 and 2006. What they found was astounding. They discovered the risk of suicide was twelve times higher and the risk of heart-related death six times higher during the first week following diagnosis compared to those who were cancer-free.

Mum initially felt overwhelmed and helpless when she discovered she had cancer. She had always dreaded the disease, and watching her brother die from leukaemia in his thirties, after a hellish year of chemo, only served to intensify that fear. 'Part of the anxiety stemmed from doubts about what I would do if I was diagnosed,' mum explains. 'I always said that I would never have chemotherapy or radiation – so what was the alternative?' But diving into cancer research and discovering myriad options put paid to mum's fear: 'When I think of cancer now I think of research, inspiring healers – I think "What more can I learn about it?"' she says.

Finding a sense of meaning amid the injustice of illness has helped many to fight the fear. When New York-based cancer counsellor and researcher Dr Kelly Turner studied those who had experienced an 'unexpected remission' of cancer, one of her subjects shared the following: 'And so instead of ever saying, "Why me?" I actually always said, "Okay, I'm listening. What am I supposed to learn here?" or "What am I supposed to teach here?"'[19]

If cancer runs in the family it's understandable you might be particularly phobic of the condition. But it's worth noting that obsessively worrying about cancer might increase your chances of getting it: 'You're going to have more lumps, bumps and trouble with your breasts, if you're focusing fear and negativity on that area,' says Dr Bernie Siegel. It's also true that staying awake at night fretting about developing the disease can compound the problem: 'Chronic insomnia is definitely present in many cancer patients,' says Dr Alexander Mostovoy. On the flip side, studies now suggest that getting enough sleep might reverse the disease: 'Although having cancer might be something to lose sleep over, we'd rather help people regain the sleep and lose the cancer,' says Dr David Spiegel.[20]

Harbouring resentment

'The very word remission, for the regression of disease, also means, according to the dictionary "relinquishing, surrendering forgiveness, pardon as of sins or crimes",' writes cancer survivor Marc Ian Barasch in his best-selling book *The Healing Path*.

We often think of forgiveness in terms of weakness: we imagine 'giving in' or 'admitting defeat' and, as a society, we tend to look down on women who take back cheating partners. But forgiveness is not necessarily about 'looking the other way'; it's actually about letting go and taking back your power.

In Dr Kelly Turner's illuminating thesis on 'unexpected remission' of cancer, one of the many healers she interviewed described forgiveness in the following way: ' ... it's a state you reach when you no longer care about it any more'.

For medical intuitive Caroline Myss, blame and forgiveness are at the heart of illness and recovery. In *Anatomy of the Spirit* she shares some thoughts on why people don't heal: 'They can't get their spirit back from the illusion that people ... have come into their lives for destructive reasons.' When your husband of twenty years suddenly ups and leaves, when an old friend betrays you or when a family member goes behind your back, anger, resentment and a need for revenge can possess you, poisoning mind and spirit and leaving you trapped in a futile quest for redemption. But if you can cultivate the compassion to forgive, you can reclaim your power and energy: 'You may get a sense that the best thing you can do is just release, the best thing you can do is just leave them alone,' writes Myss. 'Still, that is an act of divine union if you do it without hatred, if you do it without fear, if you do it without judgement.'

Caroline Myss encourages us to see how difficult relationships might help us grow. For instance, your partner's infidelity might provide you with an opportunity to meet your soul-mate; a lack of love might foster inner strength; a critical boss might help you hone your craft and remind you what it is to be humble. Of course, forgiveness also involves letting ourselves off the hook: 'Blaming oneself or someone else for an unfortunate situation results in the feeling of being a victim and is likely to manifest itself as disease,' says Andreas Moritz. 'The body stores all the experiences we have in invisible "filing cabinets". Accordingly, all the feelings of anger we have in life go into one file, sad events are placed in another and rejections are deposited in yet a different file. These impressions feed "the ghost of memory" and give it more power and energy.'

The Carcinogenic Relationship

Leading cancer specialist Dr Nicholas Gonzalez says: 'A negative, hostile, angry spouse can undermine everything I do, because the patient lives in a state of fear and anxiety.' Early on in his career, Dr Gonzalez realised that emotional health was just as important as the enzyme

▶

therapy and coffee enemas he was prescribing to patients: 'Nutrition is wonderful, but there is no vitamin, mineral or trace element that can override somebody's psychology,' he says. 'Under stress the body tissues break down to provide energy to deal with the stress – and that's the antithesis of healing.'

A prime example of the 'carcinogenic relationship' recently walked into Dr Gonzalez's office. The patient, a woman with ovarian cancer, was keen to start work with Dr Gonzalez, but her husband was clearly against it: 'He came into the room, arms folded, and within ten seconds he said, "How do I know we can trust you and that this isn't just a bunch of quackery?" and I said, "You know something? You can't know that." I then said to the patient: "You told me, your husband was supportive?" The husband left the room and his wife said to me, "He does it all the time." I didn't say this to her, but I could see right away that the main reason she had cancer was she was living with a bully.'

So can leaving a toxic relationship help you heal? The late Brendan O'Regan, former vice president of the Institute of Noetic Sciences, analysed hundreds of medical journals on the subject of 'spontaneous remission'. In his subsequent book, *Spontaneous Remission: An Annotated Bibliography*, he cites an example of a woman with metastasised cervical cancer whose health took a dramatic turn when 'her much-hated husband suddenly died, whereupon she completely recovered'.[21]

Of course, it's not only men who are to 'blame' (and let's not forget, we stay in an unhappy relationship of our own volition). Recently Dr Rashid Buttar saw a husband-and-wife team for an initial consultation: 'As we were talking,

▶

the wife interrupted her husband – who had brain cancer – not once, not twice, but three times!' says Buttar. 'Finally, I said to the wife: "When a person has a diagnosis of cancer, they are feeling helpless – like they have no control. So when you cut off your husband mid-sentence, you're taking away that little bit of control he has." The husband started laughing and said, "Don't worry Dr Buttar, my wife always does that." To me, that is why he got cancer in the first place.'

Striving for Happiness, Finding Healing

Bottom line? If depression comes from holding on to past hurts and anxiety stems from worrying about the future, perhaps a key component of staying healthy is to remain firmly in the present.

When you're faced with a serious health challenge, it might be easier to assume you're a victim of bad genes than to acknowledge that your thoughts and behaviour affect your health. By dismissing the impact of psychological factors, you can conveniently sidestep the call to change: you can hold on to old habits and leave your well-being in the hands of someone else. But ignoring the emotional aspects of cancer could be compromising your recovery, according to Dr Ruth Bolletino, New York-based psychotherapist, long-term cancer survivor and author of *How to Talk with Family Caregivers about Cancer*: 'If a cancer patient says to me, "I just want everything to be exactly as it was before I was diagnosed", that doesn't fly with me because that was the context in which the cancer grew,' she says. 'So sooner or later, we get to the question, "What in you has stopped you from finding, identifying and expressing your own best ways of living? What stops you from doing what you love?"'

Perhaps you *are* in love with your life; maybe you have already trawled the depths of self-awareness and feel in charge of your emotions. But if your soul needs nourishment, or you simply need to lower your stress levels, why not take the time to make the necessary changes? While there is no clear consensus on what causes cancer, surely it pays to leave no stone unturned? 'We do all these things to monitor our health – we do pap smears, breast exams – but how often do we really deal with the things that impact us in such a deep manner, that keep us awake at night?' asks Dr Rashid Buttar.

With groundbreaking studies being published every week demonstrating the profound power of the mind over the body, we're rapidly approaching a time when the importance of emotional health can no longer be denied in the healing paradigm. Indeed, even the Centers for Disease Control and Prevention (CDC) states that up to 90 per cent of the doctor visits in the USA may be triggered by a stress-related illness.[22] And, while there are no guarantees that letting go of toxic baggage and rediscovering lost passions will cure your cancer, it might help you find the will to live.

•

CHAPTER 3

The Cancer Survivor

*'When we are no longer able to
change a situation – we are challenged
to change ourselves.'*
Viktor E. Frankl, *Man's Search for Meaning*

Illness strikes at the heart of who you are. It casts a spell of uncertainty over every aspect of your life, leaving future plans, daily routines and often relationships in disarray. It can keep you paralysed with fear, unable to access rational thoughts or to draw from your own well of inspiration.

So when you're in that place of terror, why not look to those who have been in your shoes? While one person's route to recovery might be another's road to ruin, there is, none the less, wisdom to be gained from every patient who has walked the path to wellness and defied 'impossible' odds. In his book *The Healing Path*, Marc Ian Barasch writes eloquently about the elusive nature of recovery: 'Healing is idiosyncratic at best, a power-sharing arrangement between an individual's physiology, pathology, psyche, emotional history, social context, medicines, healer and gods. Some people I talked with went off on a quest, some stayed put, tending to their gardens; some found healing within the family, some by escaping it ...'

After speaking with hundreds of patients who, like himself,

survived a 'deadly' disease, Barasch began to see patterns emerging. He found that in many cases these remarkable individuals
were able to access an inner strength and defiance, mollify their
inner saboteur and re-evaluate their way of life: 'I began to see
my cancer as a personal message: CHANGE OR DIE,' writes
Barasch.

While it might sound flaky to talk of spirituality and inner
strength when you're faced with something as serious as cancer,
many doctors make no bones about the importance of these factors: 'If you're willing to let go and have faith, amazing things
can happen,' says cancer surgeon and best-selling author Dr
Bernie Siegel, who has devoted his life to humanising medical
care. 'People have to realise that when you have a feeling, it
affects your chemistry.' Studies show that 'positive' emotions,
like hope, are associated with the release of specific biochemicals
that have an effect on tissues and disease,[1] and while optimism
alone is unlikely to unlock the doors to healing it's nevertheless
a powerful ally. A University of Pittsburgh study found that therapy aimed at reducing cancer patients' pessimism boosted their
immune systems.[2]

Despite decades of scientific research into 'psycho-somatic'
medicine, talking about the emotional components of cancer –
and cancer recovery – still invites vehement opposition: some
critics believe those who practise mind–body medicine are placing an unnecessary burden on patients, suggesting *they* are to
blame if they don't get well. Nothing could be further from the
truth. This 'new age' paradigm is about giving patients back
power and autonomy: 'In terms of who will do well with cancer,
it's the people who see it as a challenge – more than as a threat,'
says Dr Joan Borysenko, a Harvard-trained medical scientist.
'They put their energy into things they know can make a difference, rather than trying to control the uncontrollable.'

New York psychotherapist and long-term cancer survivor Dr
Ruth Bolletino helps patients recover their zest for life: 'What is

of far more interest than the causes [of cancer] is what you can do about it,' she says. 'By changing psychological factors, you transform the total environment in which the cancer grew.'

Harness Wisdom

Since her own diagnosis mum has found psychological sustenance from therapy, workshops and a wide variety of books. From Louise Hay's positive affirmations to Thomas Moore's invitation to see illness as a 'dark night of the soul', she has taken inspiration from many teachers and looked to see where their advice might be applied to her own life. So what distinguishes the *survivor* personality? In this chapter we shine a light on seven pieces of the healing puzzle:

Find your J-spot

Sitting on the Eurostar, halfway across the English Channel mum turned to me and said: 'I'm going to enjoy myself this weekend.' I shot her back a quizzical look. 'I'm going to have a croissant if I feel like it, maybe a glass of champagne, so don't get angry with me,' she cautioned. Given that mum had spent more than a year drinking green juice, cutting out sugar, dairy and gluten and doing coffee enemas, I figured she could afford to let her wimples down for a weekend (and the frozen wheatgrass shots I'd insisted on taking to Paris would surely protect against a few pastries).

But for some alternative cancer travellers, pleasure is a foreign land. They never eat out, for fear of unwittingly consuming a quenelle of cream; they won't travel abroad ('Haven't you heard of cosmic radiation?') and 'down time' means spending hours in seated meditation. Don't get me wrong; many survivors credit their recovery to daily contemplation and a strict diet. But if every waking hour is taken up with activities that make your heart sink, then perhaps it's time for an injection of Joy: perhaps you need to rediscover your J-spot.

'When people don't have any excitement or enthusiasm in their lives, it's just not healthy,' says Dr Ruth Bolletino. Andreas Moritz, author of *Cancer is Not a Disease: It's a Survival Mechanism* has a similar view: 'When you are too puritanical about any-thing – even if it's conducive to good health – you are still living in a state of anxiety, a state of fear ... True healing is about living a natural, healthy, balanced life. One where you are doing things that give you pleasure.'

The good news is that doing something purely for enjoyment can protect you from harm. In the mid-1990s, Dr Lee Berk of Loma Linda University in California found that laughter actually increases the number of natural killer cells in cancer patients (these immune cells play a major role in scuppering tumours). More recent research suggests a good giggle can be as beneficial as exercise. According to an article in the *Telegraph*, 'Doctors describe "mirthful laughter" as the equivalent of "internal jog-ging" because it can lower blood pressure, stress and boost the immune system much like moderate exercise.'[3] Pleasure is pow-erful stuff. In fact, having a sense of joy is the second most important factor for predicting cancer survival, according to research from Sandra Levy, associate professor of psychiatry and medicine at the University of Pittsburgh.[4]

Feeling euphoric also provides free access to Interleukin-2. The synthetic version of the substance – the cancer drug Proleukin – costs around $40,000 and comes with a long list of side effects.[5] But according to medical research you can boost your own secretions of Interleukin-2 just by being relaxed and joyful. Dr Ursula Jacob, one of Germany's leading oncologists, explains that Interleukin-2 receptors are 'always low' in cancer patients, so there's even more reason to make time for leisure.

It sounds so simple. But is it really? One in three British work-ers fails to take their full annual holiday entitlement according to a recent survey.[6] Instead they put in 36 million hours of free overtime. The relentless pressures of twenty-first-century life mean many of us have forgotten what it means to 'let go'. Cancer patients often ask Toronto-based physician Dr Alexander Mostovoy what they should do to relax: 'I encourage patients to remember a time when they were little – perhaps being totally absorbed playing with a doll – when nothing else existed and they had no care. It's about finding that feeling again, that's your place of healing,' says Mostovoy.

Finding pleasure and fulfilment is a key component of Dr Bernie Siegel's workshops for Exceptional Cancer Patients (ECaP): '"Do I have enough play in my life?" That's what patients need to ask themselves,' he says. 'So finding things that help you lose track of time. Because then you're in a trance state, and that's the healthiest state to be in.'

When Rachel Kierath was diagnosed with an aggressive breast cancer at the age of thirty-one, she decided to live 'decadently': 'I gave up my [teaching] position, which, as a single parent at that point was a scary prospect, but I decided to just focus on myself which was such a wonderful indulgence,' says Rachel. 'I guess it [cancer] freed up the time for me to focus on all the things in life – like preparing healthy food, exercise, meditation – that we know we should do, but we don't.'

Escape the 'lovely' trap

If you constantly override your own basic needs to look after others', you might be suffering from what psychologist Jacqui Marson refers to as the 'curse of lovely': 'In my fifteen years of clinical experience I have seen many women and men's lives – relationships, careers and wellbeing – blighted by the belief they have to be a "lovely person" in order to be accepted,' says Marson, author of *The Curse of Lovely*. 'This might mean always being polite, helpful, charming, fun, making people feel good about themselves, not letting people down, avoiding conflict and putting others' needs before their own.'

Sound familiar? Marson's description of the 'lovely' bears a striking resemblance to the 'cancer personality' (see Chapter 2). Whether or not you believe these traits are carcinogenic, there's little doubt that continually putting others first can undermine your sense of worth and zap your energy. But is it really possible to break decades-old behaviour patterns?

'I often ask clients: what would one per cent different look like?' says Marson. 'So rather than attacking the big life changes like, "Do I leave my husband?" or "Should I quit my job?" you might start thinking about how to respond to the moment-to-moment choices throughout your day.' You might, for example, decide not to engage in a conversation with a woman on the tube, or say 'No' to lunch with a needy colleague. 'When you recognise that "this person is actually making a demand on me", then you have the power to decide whether to give away your energy or not,' says Marson.

In *The Curse of Lovely* the reader is invited to 'disappoint someone daily': 'Believe it or not, there are people out there who, when asked to the temporary receptionist's birthday drinks, just say, "Sorry, I would love to, but I really can't make it" with a gracious smile and no guilt,' she says. The art of the 'gracious no', according to Marson, involves sandwiching your polite refusal between two positive statements. 'So for instance, you might say, "Thank you for thinking of me, I'll have to pass on that this time, but I would love to meet up in a few months when work is less busy." If you can't decide on the spot, simply say, "I need to check with my diary first",' she suggests.

Learning to say no doesn't mean morphing into a cold-hearted monster, assures Marson; it's about finding the middle ground. When faced with a situation that requires assertiveness, Marson likes to think of her Danish friend Mette: 'Mette's straightforwardness was a revelation to me. A few years ago my family went to stay with hers. Within an hour of arriving she looked me in the eye and said: "We have just had people staying and I am sick of cooking, so I will not be cooking for you. There are lots of places to eat out and please help yourselves to anything in the kitchen." We ended up having a great time and it was largely because there was a very relaxed atmosphere with no undercurrents of resentment or tension seeping out like poison gas from our hostess.'

Constantly putting others first might be the mark of a saint, but more often than not, it's a sign of low self-esteem. If you don't believe your needs are as important as those around you, then it might be time for some self-love.

Boost your self-worth

Caroline Myss, medical intuitive and best-selling author, believes self-esteem is the fundamental power of life. 'I have discovered in my years of work that people with low self-esteem do not heal with the speed or as deeply as people who have healthy self-esteem,' she says in her audio-book *Self-Esteem: Your Fundamental Power*. Many practitioners (and patients) are bound to be enraged by this perspective. To tell someone who is already suffering from low self-worth that they're sabotaging their efforts to get well can seem like a particularly low blow. None the less, many long-term cancer survivors stress that looking after their emotional health has been vital to their recovery.

For those who are cynical of the self-help message to 'love yourself', rest assured – boosting confidence needn't involve scribbling positive messages on the bathroom mirror or identifying the beauty in your little fingernail; it's about making changes in your life and taking action. 'Building self-esteem ... is a step-by-step, brick-by-brick process in which you target your deficits,' says Myss. Just as a budding entrepreneur would take time to analyse where he's losing money, Myss urges us to be aware of situations that are draining our power. You might, for example, notice you 'try a bit hard' when you're with an old school friend or feel resentment rising when your partner cuts you off mid-sentence. Whenever you sense you're abdicating power or not being true to yourself, notice it and imagine how you might respond differently.

Alternatively, you could focus on areas in your life where you *do* feel in control: 'Today the term "low self-esteem" feels very critical; it can imply failure,' says Marson. 'I encourage clients to look for exceptions to that rule, to identify situations where they *do* feel confident. It's important for people to recognise that everyone has that strong side.'

Reading self-help books, keeping a journal or seeing a therapist can all bring about new insights which foster self-compassion. Sometimes we need to see something written on a page or hear ourselves speak the words aloud to fully understand the way we feel. But awareness is not enough, according to Caroline Myss. She believes action is also critical: 'You've got to become a verb and not a noun,' she emphasises in *Self-Esteem*. 'Verbs heal, nouns don't ... Whatever skill you have, you have got to wake it up and put it in motion.'

Exercise is a simple way to clear your mind, boost your confidence and activate your body's healing potential. In October 2000 researchers from Duke University made headlines[7] with a study showing that exercise is better than the drug Zoloft (or Lustral in the UK) at treating depression. 'I tell people that going for a run is like taking a little bit of Prozac and a little bit of Ritalin because, like the drugs, exercise elevates these neurotransmitters,' writes Dr John Ratey in *Spark! How Exercise will Improve the Performance of your Brain*. Exercise has also been shown to reduce cancer recurrence by up to 50 per cent according to recent studies. One study, published in 2005 from Harvard Medical School, found that women who walked one to three hours a week at a moderate pace had a 20 per cent reduced risk of breast cancer death. Among women who walked three to five hours a week, the risk was reduced by 50 per cent.[8]

Here we see the dynamic interplay of illness, emotions and recovery. The research reinforces the idea that when you revitalise your body, it has a knock-on effect on your mind – and vice versa.

Be a difficult patient

'To be a "good" patient means to be docile and fit in and do what the system wants,' writes Dr Bernie Siegel in *Peace, Love and Healing*. 'But that is not good for survival.' Siegel encourages patients to take inspiration from the word 'curious' for survival tips: '"curious" has the same root as "cure", and that means that doctors should be glad when patients come in with a list of questions, a request for options and an insistence on knowing how they can participate in their own healing.'

However, the reality of the patient/doctor relationship often falls short of this utopian vision. Having endured the rigours of medical school, many doctors find it galling when patients question their professional advice: 'My local GP tried very hard to persuade me to have surgery,' says Jane Wallis, who was diagnosed with advanced bladder cancer eight years ago. 'As he was talking I glimpsed a copy of a letter I had sent to the surgeon on his computer, explaining the reasons I didn't want to have my bladder and most of my kidney removed. I saw that the surgeon had scrawled all over the letter with rude comments. One remark that I remember vividly was: "Who does this bloody woman think she is?" When the doctor realised I could see it he switched the computer off very quickly. That was the last time I went in any doctor's surgery. It only took eight months for my body to be 100 per cent cured after starting to take apricot kernels and I've been well since then.' (See Chapter 12 for more about this story.)

Whether you follow conventional advice or choose your own way, it's important you voice your needs and ask for the best treatment for you. A recent survey found that British cancer patients were 'dying of politeness' and that those who refused to take no for an answer had a better chance of survival.[9] 'Too many people say, "Yes doctor, no doctor, three bags full doctor",' says Professor Jane Plant, author of *Your Life in Your Hands*.[10] 'Instead they should make it clear they want to be fully involved in decisions.' Plant was diagnosed with breast cancer in 1987. Despite a radical mastectomy, thirty-five radiotherapy treatments and chemotherapy the cancer kept coming back. The final time, when a malignant lump appeared on her neck, the doctors told her there was little they could do. But Plant, like many cancer survivors, refused to accept the medical verdict. Instead she embarked on a dedicated research campaign, which led to her discovery that dairy was the root cause of her disease (see Chapter 8).

This 'fighting spirit' is echoed in many cancer survivor stories, and research suggests it can indeed aid recovery. One study published in the *Lancet* looked at fifty-seven women diagnosed with early breast cancer. After ten years, the research revealed that 70 per cent of those with 'fighting spirit' were still alive, as opposed to 20 per cent of those who reacted to their diagnoses with hopelessness and helplessness.[11] Bernie Siegel has coined the term 'respant' to describe 'responsible participants': patients who aren't afraid to get involved and rock the boat. 'They fight the submissive role because they are fighting for their lives, so I naturally encourage them in that behaviour,' writes Dr Siegel in *Peace, Love and Healing*. 'The result is that my patients tend to get reputations.'

In *Cancer as a Turning Point*, Dr Lawrence LeShan cautions against being a compliant patient: 'While the meek may inherit the earth, unless you are in a hurry to inherit your six feet of it, do not be meek.' Refusing to lie down quietly can make you unpopular, but it also can help you heal. Researchers from Yale found there was a direct correlation between an active immune system and a negative opinion of the patient by the head nurse on the ward.[12]

But being a survivor needn't mean going into a ward with a verbal battle-axe. Assertiveness, rather than rudeness, is what's called for when your life is on the line. In *The Healing Path* Marc Barasch recounts the story of one long-term survivor who refused to accept her terminal diagnosis. When the first doctor she saw handed her a book called *Good Grief* Annie Nathan decided to look further afield. When she finally found a doctor she admired, she said to him: 'I'm not going to hold you responsible for what happens to me. But I'm holding tryouts for my healing team and I want to know if you want to be on it.'

Find fulfilment

Do you have any regrets? Would you have done things differently? These are the questions Bronnie Ware, an Australian nurse, asked patients in the years she spent working in palliative care. Ware noticed common themes surfacing again and again and she eventually put her observations into a book called *The Top Five Regrets of the Dying*. So what was the number-one regret, as recorded by Ware? 'I wish I'd had the courage to live a life true to myself, not the life others expected of me.'

Mum now admits that prior to her diagnosis she had lost her passion for life. She had forgone a career to look after four children, but when we finally left home she was left stymied with indecision. A full-time job seemed a lofty goal after two decades out of the workforce; and as for a hobby, she had considered writing and photography courses, but nothing really sparked her fire. Mum felt the insistent nudge of dissatisfaction, yet the fear of being judged stayed her hand.

But there's nothing like cancer to ring the alarm bells. In the early 1900s the Jungian analyst Elida Evans described cancer as 'growth gone wrong' and 'a message to take a new road in your life' and that's just what mum did. She stopped navel gazing and started speaking about her experience – on the radio, at seminars – spreading the word about alternative cancer treatments and responding to the requests for more information which streamed into her inbox daily.

In shamanic culture there are various spiritual explanations for disease: it may result from a loss of animal spirit guides, 'loss of soul' or 'when the patient has special talents he does or does not use'.[13] This focus on 'what is missing' in a patient's life contrasts sharply with Western medicine's preoccupation with what the patient 'has got' in terms of disease. Traditional psychotherapy follows this Western model, aiming to unearth the root cause of a patient's presenting problem.

Dr Lawrence LeShan, regarded as the pioneer of cancer psychology, offers a different approach through his innovative therapy. As Dr Ruth Bolletino, who has worked alongside LeShan for over two decades, explains: 'The first question we ask is not "What's wrong with the person?" but "What's right with the person?" We identify what vitalises the person and look at what can be added or changed in their life to make it more fulfilling. We also consider goals or dreams he or she might want to pursue and what steps the person might take to begin moving in that direction.' So how effective is this radical approach? While Bolletino has not kept a statistical record of survivors – 'the clients I see have different kinds and stages of cancer, and different kinds of medical and complementary treatment, so the statistics would be meaningless' – she does concede that the cancer patients she treats continually 'exceed medical expectations'. Over the past thirty years that he has been practising psychotherapy, approximately half of LeShan's cancer patients with poor prognoses have experienced long-term remission and many are still alive.

Deborah[14] is a striking example of someone who surpassed a dire prognosis through living her dreams. Twenty years ago Deborah was diagnosed with stage-4 ovarian cancer: she had hoped to become a successful dancer, but was instead told she had months to live. 'So she moved to another country, opened a holistic health centre, became a successful dance therapist and now, twenty years later, quips that "Dancing became stage five",' says Bolletino.

So what stops us from finding fulfilment – the supposed jewel in the healing crown? 'I've seen many clients over the years who come to me feeling "stuck",' says Jacqui Marson. 'Often, they hate their job or they're unhappy in their relationship and they can't seem to see a way out.' Ironically, being miserable can blind you to other options: 'If you are doing something that's making you unhappy, you can feel very crushed by that, and the resilient, problem-solving parts of yourself become frozen.' Marson encourages clients to find an activity or ritual that provides the opportunity to experiment with change: 'For some people it's signing up for an exercise class they have never dared to walk into, for others it's literally cooking a new recipe and discovering that, even if it's a failure, they are okay.'

Many people feel trapped in jobs that run counter to who they really are. While doing something you can't stand day in day out is almost certainly going to affect your health, simply handing in your notice is not always an option. Marson instead urges clients to explore other possibilities while staying in their existing job: 'Often just going to a recruitment agent and discovering you are eligible for other jobs makes you feel more empowered,' says Marson. 'So you might decide to stay in the old job, but no longer take the same c**p from your boss,' she says. 'The answer might be the same for your relationship: once you feel fulfilled, it can change the dynamic completely.'

Fight fear

At a recent London workshop, Caroline Myss posed the rhetorical question: 'Why do I anticipate the worst when time and time again the worst never happens?' All of us can recall instances when fear has fuelled catastrophic fantasies: we imagine the dog has been run over, our child has been taken, that rash is really meningitis – and yet everything has turned out okay. But when that creeping feeling of apprehension overcomes us, we tend to think only of worst-case scenarios. 'When we encounter something that makes us feel anxious, it sets off the amygdala, an almond-shaped mass located deep within the temporal lobe of the brain which is like a car alarm,' says Jacqui Marson. 'Adrenaline floods your body, gearing you up to run, fight or freeze and your conscious thinking brain is blocked.'

Fear can also send your immune system on strike: 'The digestive system doesn't function when you are worried and anxious, so you don't make enough bile and pancreatic enzymes – vital for cancer patients,' says Andreas Moritz. 'Under those circumstances, it's very difficult for the body to heal.' Dr Bernie Siegel offers a similar warning: 'If all you do is live in fear, then your body can't heal and grow.'

Yet recognising the destructive potential of fear does little to soothe the soul. Many cancer patients find themselves caught in a cycle of dread and despair, where they worry about the cancer, and then worry about worrying: 'I urge my clients not to beat themselves up about any feelings they might have,' says Dr Ruth Bolletino. 'Anyone diagnosed with cancer goes through storms of emotions: shock, disbelief, fear, anxiety, anger, frustration, grief, despair, even guilt. And anyone who has had cancer fears recurrence for a long time afterwards as I know from my own experience.'

Rachel Kiereth, who defied a grim cancer prognosis through nutrition and herbal supplements, describes how she conquered the fear: 'There is so much hype and fear surrounding cancer, so I had to kind of process that as quickly as I could,' she says. 'I had to just say to myself: "Stop! You know there are so many other options out there." So I went back to what I knew and what I had researched.' (See Chapter 12 for more about this story.)

When New York-based cancer counsellor Dr Kelly Turner quizzed those who had experienced an 'unexpected remission' from cancer, she found that letting go of fear, and particularly the fear of death, was cited frequently.

So while fear might be natural for cancer patients, there *are* ways to avoid being a slave to the emotion. Some experts favour the reverse psychology approach of building fifteen minutes of 'worry time' into your day, the idea being that when forced to worry, you might find that doubts and distress evaporate. You could also try transforming panic into a positive energy, which worked for ex-anxiety sufferer Charles Linden, creator of the Linden Method. After attending a four-day Linden Method retreat, the writer William Leith described his new-found insight in a magazine article: 'At the end I feel uplifted . . . I see that going round in circles, worrying, is much less interesting than, say, getting up early in the morning and writing books. I see that it is possible to replace my pernicious worry with a sort of excitement.'[15]

Dr Ruth Bolletino encourages patients to swap anxiety for anticipation: 'They have to know there's an exciting future waiting for them afterwards,' she says. 'I urge them to start making plans – big ones, small ones – things they can look forward to which remind them of who they are and that they have a future.'[16]

Fear often stems from the unfamiliar or unknown, but talking to those who have been there, and survived, can provide reassurance. When Dr Bernie Siegel invited a ninety-year-old woman to join his support group she put people's fears in perspective: 'Because she had lived through every damned thing everyone else is so afraid of.'

Making room for spirituality has helped mum, and many others, navigate the dark nights. But prayer isn't for everyone. 'For people who are agnostic or atheist, being spiritual may mean going for a walk in the late evening and feeling the vastness of the night sky,' says Joshua Rosenthal, founder and director of the Institute for Integrative Nutrition in the US. 'It has been my experience that when people feel connected with the big picture, they get healthier faster.'

Just drop it

Mum quickly discovered that her cancer diagnosis was an open invitation for psycho-spiritual advice: 'Often ovarian cancer is to do with unresolved issues surrounding relationships,' said one practitioner, whom she consulted for advice on ozone (see Chapter 9). 'Well if that is the case, how do I let go of these "issues"'? mum asked. 'It's not that easy.'

'Really?' the doctor replied. With that, he picked a book up from the table and held it in the air. Looking mum straight in the eye, he said, 'I don't really want to hold on to this book, but how do I get rid of it?' He paused, before dropping the book on the floor. 'Oh, that's right, it is easy: you just drop it.'

While some people possess the strength of character to single-handedly exorcise their demons, many more seek the help of therapists and healers. Mum found solace in a motorbike-riding psychologist, reiki master and Traditional Chinese Medical Practitioner called Casey Terry. Using a combination of techniques, Terry helps clients to unearth and release unresolved stress and traumas. 'I look for the core disruption in the flow of energy,' Terry explains. 'The brain stores trauma in the amygdala – the emotional brain – and it keeps running that trauma in the body, like a CD on repeat. That leads to emotional blockages – usually in the tissues, muscles or tendons.'

For those in doubt, this is not fringe theory: it's frontier medicine. Thanks to discoveries in quantum physics and molecular biology we now know a great deal about the energetic basis of thought and its connection to our physical well-being (see Chapter 11). Dr Bernie Siegel explains the link in more scientific terms: 'There are approximately sixty known peptide molecules in the body, including some with names that may be familiar to you, like endorphins, interleukins and interferon. They make feelings chemical.' It's these chemicals that link body and mind. Dr Bradley Nelson, author of the groundbreaking book *The Emotion Code*, writes that trapped emotions 'can interfere with proper function of your body's organs and tissues, wreaking havoc with your physical health causing pain, fatigue and illness'.

So what's the answer? One-to-one therapy, tapping, NLP, energy healing, or simply putting pen to paper can all help to release toxic baggage; indeed, studies show that people who record traumatic experiences in a diary show better immune function.[17] In Dr Bernie Siegel's workshops participants are often handed paper and crayons to help resolve dilemmas and gain personal insight: 'The unconscious speaks through dreams and drawings,' explains Siegel, 'so you might discover what's eating away at someone or what's missing in their lives,' he says.

Dr Rashid A. Buttar, renowned physician, detox expert and author of *The 9 Steps to Keep the Doctor Away*, believes cancer is always triggered by a psychological trauma or unresolved issue: 'I see it all the time in my practice, even with patients who seem, on the surface, to be trouble-free,' he says. One of the first things Dr Buttar asks his cancer patients to do is to write down a list of people who owe them an apology: 'Whether they're alive or not, it doesn't matter,' says Buttar, 'but whoever has done you wrong – whoever has left you with a hurt you're still holding on to – write that person's name down, then forgive them.' Buttar stresses the act of forgiving must be meaningful: 'It's not just simply saying, "I forgive you", but truly letting go. You're not forgiving them because they deserve forgiveness; you're forgiving them because *you* deserve to be free of carrying that burden.'

Your Road Map to Healing

When dealing with cancer it's important to remember there is no 'one-size-fits-all' approach: you can look to survivors for inspiration, but ultimately the answer lies in identifying what *your* mind and body are lacking.

In *The Healing Path* Marc Barasch describes sitting quietly and talking to his cancer: '"Why have you come?" I asked loudly, feeling unutterably silly. "Can't live this way," I heard the voice rasp with great bitterness.' Not many patients will try this unusual technique, but the idea really resonated with mum: 'So I did that. I sat quietly with my cancer and I thought, "Why have you come?" I had led such a "healthy" physical life – I'd exercised, I'd eaten organic ... but the answer really screamed back at me: "You have no joy in your life! You always have this really big to-do list, but where is your joy?" I had looked after my physical health, but I had really neglected my emotional health,' says mum.

In the eyes of Dr Leonard Coldwell, a leading cancer specialist and authority on stress-related illness, it's more important to identify the root cause of cancer than to remove the tumour: 'You have to understand that it will never be one single thing that cures cancer,' he says. 'If you get vitamin C intravenously, three times a day for twelve days, your cancerous tumours – in my experience – will disappear. But of course they will come back if you never address the root cause: the bad marriage, the horrible job, the constantly making compromises against yourself, the lack of hope, the lack of love, the lack of self-love. These are the causes of cancer.'

Dr Coldwell has developed the Instinct Based Medicine

System™ – a series of audio CDs aimed at helping the patient identify and eliminate the root cause of their illness. The recordings feature unique sound frequencies, which allegedly penetrate deep into the brainwaves of the patient. 'I need to have you in beta waves when I want you to make a decision; alpha waves if I want you to be passive and I need to have you in theta or delta waves if I want you to heal,' explains Coldwell.

There are, of course, many methods for gaining insight into your illness and acquiring peace of mind – meditation, journaling and energy healing – to name just a few. But whatever tools you use, it's important to follow through with positive action. 'Just sitting there, reciting positive affirmations and expecting some magic force to cure you will not work,' says Dr Leonard Coldwell. 'You need to take charge and take responsibility for your own life.' So imagining your body cloaked in healing light won't do much good if you're filling it with burgers and fries.

Moving from the passive role of victim to that of cancer victor can take a variety of forms. You might work on building your self-worth and start saying 'No', you might find the courage to pursue your fantasy job or you might simply decide to prioritise spending more time outdoors, growing a garden and nurturing your spirit. But whatever you do, expect good things. You never hear of people overdosing on 'hope' or dying as a result of radical change.

'The key, in my experience, is trust,' writes Barasch. 'Trust is an implicit, deep faith that leaves no room for doubt or scepticism. "I believe this will work" is not trust's end point; rather, trust's starting point is "I *know* this will work".'

CHAPTER 4

•

Vitamin Injections

*'Vitamin C is one of my top choices
as an alternative to chemo.'*
Dr Norm Shealy, neurosurgeon, psychologist and
founder of the American Holistic Medical Association

Long before mum became a cancer research buff, she was known as the go-to woman for anti-ageing advice. Friends and family would quiz mum on beauty creams, exercise trends and age-defying supplements and she would eagerly share the latest news from the front. Anything she read about that promised to turn back the clock was given a go, no matter how wacky it sounded.

For years she kept kombucha – a jellyfish-like culture – in a pot on the kitchen worktop. She drank the juice and occasionally, when the mood would take her, she'd whizz the gelatinous lump in a blender and use it on her face. Then there was the headstand machine (the ultimate way to defy gravity), the anti-ageing mouth guard and the laser hair combs, reported to restore hair to its youthful lustre. Mum even tried vitamin injections a couple of times. She had read they could revitalise the body and increase longevity and, with the likes of Cindy Crawford touting their benefits, she wanted in on the action. Little did mum know how valuable the treatment would be for her years later, or how lucky she was to know where to get her fix.

Recent research and films like the revolutionary documentary *Food Matters* have raised the profile of this powerful healing therapy and roused the interest of cancer patients who might not otherwise have been into alternatives. The only problem is finding a practitioner. Indeed, the question I'm asked most frequently on my blog from readers all over the world is: 'Where can I get vitamin C injections?'

So what is vitamin C therapy? 'Instead of treating cancer with chemotherapy, you can give intravenous vitamin C at, 30,000, 60,000, 100,000 milligrams a day, directly into the bloodstream and that will kill cancer cells. With vitamin C, there is no damage to healthy cells,' explains health educator and author Dr Andrew Saul in *Food Matters*. The documentary provides a whirlwind tour of everything that's wrong with our food chain – from genetically modified corn to the cost of healthy food – and looks at what we can do to restore our world to health. The cancer epidemic is put under the spotlight and cutting-edge therapies like vitamin C injections are discussed in detail.

Serendipitously, mum happened to have watched the film three weeks prior to her diagnosis, so as soon as she left hospital, she made a beeline for the doctor who she knew offered 'drip' vitamins. She started having 60,000 milligrams of vitamin C intravenously (IVC), twice to three times a week. To give you some idea of just how much this is, the recommended dietary allowance is a paltry 120mg. 'That is the amount recommended to ensure you don't get scurvy,' explains Professor Ian Brighthope, a medical doctor and surgeon and Australia's leading expert in nutritional medicine. 'It's not the dose for optimal health.'

Professor Brighthope has been treating patients with IV vitamin C for over thirty-five years. In the past, as the leader and president of the Nutritional and Environmental Medicine College, he was attacked relentlessly by members of his own profession for his 'controversial' views and therapies. By 1980 he'd had enough, after being fined $5000 and wrongly found guilty of professional misconduct for writing a book about nutrition and speaking out about diet and vitamins in relation to serious disease. He took on the Medical Board of Victoria in a Supreme Court trial and won. The Medical Board was reprimanded and Professor Brighthope subsequently supported large numbers of doctors who were charged with professional misconduct for using nutrients and diet in therapy.

So how did Professor Brighthope first hear about intravenous vitamin C? 'I had some clues from Linus Pauling in the US, but I basically taught myself,' said Brighthope. 'I used vitamin C experimentally in a cancer patient who was terminal – and the patient lived for another seven years.'

Where It All Began

More than forty years ago, Dr Linus Pauling (twice Nobel prize winner and associate of Einstein) and Dr Ewan Cameron conducted a number of studies looking at the effect of vitamin C therapy in cancer patients. In 1971, 100 terminal cancer patients were given 10g (10,000mg) of vitamin C intravenously a day, compared to a control group of 1000 patients who were treated by conventional methods only.

Five years after the beginning of the study, 18 of the 100 vitamin C-treated patients were still living while all 1000 of the control patients had died.[1]

Since then there has been an explosion of research into vitamin C and cancer. In 1991 Dr Gladys Block, formerly with the National Cancer Institute (NCI) in the USA, published an exhaustive review of research on vitamin C. Dr Block concluded: 'Approximately 90 epidemiologic studies have examined the role of vitamin C or vitamin-C-rich foods in cancer prevention and the vast majority have found statistically significant protective effects. Evidence is strong for cancers of the oesophagus, oral cavity, stomach and pancreas. There is also substantial evidence of a protective effect in cancers of the cervix, rectum and breast. Even in lung cancer ... there is recent evidence of a role for vitamin C.'[2]

There's good news for those with uterine cancer too. A study from Japan found that those suffering from the condition lived fifteen times longer if they were having intravenous vitamin C.[3] Not surprisingly, low levels of vitamin C are thought to contribute to the risk of uterine cancer. In 2010 New Zealand researchers compared normal tissue and malignant tissue taken from women with cancer of the uterus. They found that high-grade tumours had around 40 per cent less vitamin C than normal tissue.[4] The report appeared in a journal published by the American Association for Cancer Research (AACR).[5] Since 1980, numerous studies have reported that vitamin C is also toxic to melanoma cells.[6] In fact, melanoma seems to be more susceptible to vitamin C toxicity than any other malignancy.[7]

Leading health organisations, including the National Institutes of Health[8] in America, are now getting behind the research: 'Today we're seeing certain insurance companies in America actually pay for high-dose vitamin C for cancer patients,' says Dr Thomas Lodi, an integrative oncologist based in Arizona.

A Dangerous Fad?

The hysteria that often attends talk of high-dose vitamins has no basis in reality. 'The biggest myth about vitamin C injections is that they're dangerous,' says Dr Wendy Denning, a London-based practitioner who has been treating patients with intravenous vitamins for fifteen years. 'In all my time I have never seen a serious reaction to intravenous vitamin C. I have had a few people get faint during the infusion or develop discomfort in their veins;

some have felt tired that day ... but generally speaking, the reactions are very mild and certainly not dangerous.' So no chance of overdosing then? 'Vitamin C is water soluble, meaning your body can't store it, so any excess in your blood is expelled through your urine,' Dr Denning explains.

Patrick Holford, one of Britain's leading nutritionists and author of *Say No to Cancer*, urges people to look beyond the sensationalist headlines: 'Almost everyone has heard rumours that high-dose vitamin C causes kidney stones or might interfere with other cancer treatments. But these are only rumours. Vitamin C has been extensively studied for its potential to cause kidney stones, and it doesn't. Even the British Government's Expert Report on Vitamins and Minerals accepts this.'

The benefits of IVC for cancer patients are numberless, according to Holford: 'Vitamin C is believed to help prevent and treat cancer by enhancing the immune system; stimulating the formation of collagen which is necessary for "walling off" tumours; preventing metastasis; preventing viruses that can cause cancer; correcting a vitamin C deficiency which is often seen in cancer patients; speeding up wound healing after surgery; enhancing the effectiveness of some chemotherapy drugs; reducing the toxicity of some chemotherapy; preventing free radical damage and neutralising some carcinogens.'

When you consider the risks involved with taking pharmaceutical drugs, it seems laughable to worry about vitamins. Dr Mark Hyman, an international authority on functional medicine, underscored this paradox in a recent article for the *Huffington Post*: 'Unfortunately negative studies on vitamins get huge media attention, while the fact that over 100,000 Americans die and 2.2 million suffer serious adverse reactions from medication use in hospitals when used as prescribed is quietly ignored. Did you know that anti-inflammatories like aspirin and ibuprofen kill more people every year than AIDS or asthma or leukemia?'[9]

Don't Forget Vitamin D!

Growing up in Perth, Australia, the one thing guaranteed to make mum see red was getting burned. 'You'll get skin cancer,' she would fume as we walked in the door beetroot-coloured, after spending the day at the beach. But now it seems mum's paranoia – mirrored by mothers and government agencies globally – was way overblown.

'Most people believe that exposure to sunlight increases their risk of cancer,' says integrative oncologist Dr Thomas Lodi. 'This is simply not true. In fact, insufficient sun exposure is an important risk factor in the development of many cancers in both Western Europe and North America according to a study published in March of 2002 in the journal, *Cancer*.'

Staying out of the sun diminishes our levels of vitamin D and low levels are linked to everything from multiple sclerosis and diabetes to obesity[10] *and* cancer. There are now over 800 fully referenced studies demonstrating vitamin D's effectiveness for cancer prevention,[11] and adequate levels have been shown to reduce metastasis, increase apoptosis (programmed cell death) and double the survival rates of colorectal cancer patients.[12]

St George's Hospital in London deduced from their studies that women with low levels of vitamin D in their breast tissue have a 354 per cent greater risk of breast cancer.[13] Other studies have shown that optimal levels of vitamin D might prevent sixteen different types of cancer[14] including pancreatic, lung, ovarian, prostate and skin cancers. 'It is as if vitamin D turns cancer cells OFF!' says Dr Lodi. 'This is why we see the prevalence of cancer so low for populations of people who live on, or near the equator

▶

and a steady increase in that prevalence the further north or south one goes.'

You might assume working outdoors would leave you more vulnerable to skin cancer, but research suggests it's actually office workers who need to worry: 'When you look at scientific studies you find that skin cancer occurs mostly in people who are never exposed to the sun,' says Andreas Moritz, author of *Cancer is Not a Disease – It's A Survival Mechanism*. 'They are often people who get up in the morning at 7am to go to the office, work indoors under artificial lighting and who come home at 7pm: they never see the sun.'

So how much sun is enough?

Dr Lodi recommends one half hour of full exposure to intense natural sunlight on a near-daily basis with no sunscreen. 'This is important for vibrational nutrition and essential for mental health, bone density [and] vitamin D production,' he says. The dminder app for iPhone tells you when the sun is at the right angle to provide you with adequate vitamin D.

When mum was diagnosed with cancer, her blood levels of vitamin D were extremely low. She immediately ditched the sunscreen and started spending more time in the garden and on the beach. She also started taking vitamin D3 in spray form, following expert advice.

The daily dose

Worldwide estimates suggest that 1 billion people have inadequate levels of vitamin D in their blood.[15] So should

▶

we all be supplementing? Requirements for the sunshine vitamin are highly individual and your heritage, work environment and innate ability to produce vitamin D all play a role, so it's important to get tested before you start taking high doses. If you decide to go down that road, there are a few points you might want to consider. Firstly, take vitamin D with good-quality fats – think fish, olive and coconut oils, avocados – as this will help with absorption. Secondly, it's vital to take the right kind; doctors typically prescribe synthetic vitamin D2 – the form you'll find in fortified milk and cereal products – but it may not be absorbed as well. Research shows that vitamin D3 (a more natural form) is 87 per cent more effective than vitamin D2 at raising and maintaining vitamin D levels.[16] Taking too much vitamin D can be toxic to the liver, according to Andreas Moritz, but the good news is you can't overdose on sunshine: 'If you're in the sun for eight or ten hours – the UVA rays will break down any excess vitamin D,' he explains.

Can you get vitamin D from food?

Experts agree that it isn't easy to get enough vitamin D from your diet.[17] However, a few good dietary sources include shiitake mushrooms, eggs and oily fish. 'Sardines are one of the best foods containing vitamin D. One small tin of sardines will provide you with approximately 70 per cent of your daily needs,'[18] says Dr Edward Group, a natural health educator and cancer research expert.

In the perpetually grey-skied UK you can now find a little piece of Miami hidden away on Harley Street. The

▶

Wholistic Medical Centre (and indeed a growing number of spas and wellness facilities around the country) now offers 'Real Sunlight' treatment. For around £50 you can recline on a sun lounger and soak up the 'natural sunlight' provided by Swedish 'sunlight stimulators'. Of course, at that price, a trip to Barcelona might be a cheaper option.

Iain Chalmers, director of the UK Cochrane Centre (part of the NHS Research & Development Programme), has said that, 'Critics of complementary medicine often seem to operate a double standard, being far more assiduous in their attempts to outlaw unevaluated complementary medical practices than unevaluated orthodox practices . . . '[19] Since the listed side effects of certain chemotherapy drugs include heart attack, stroke and cancer, you may well wonder why they are not subjected to the same level of scrutiny. 'In time I think we will find that oncology is just as bad, if not worse in the scientific age, as bloodletting, as giving an amputation without an anaesthetic, as doing some of the very, very dangerous things that we used to do in medicine,' says Professor Brighthope.

Vitamin C and Chemotherapy

Patients having chemotherapy are often cautioned against having vitamin C therapy for fear it will interfere with their treatment. Professor Brighthope believes this is nonsense: 'Intravenous vitamin C reduces the toxic effects of chemotherapy, accelerates the healing after chemotherapy and reduces the inflammation caused by radiotherapy,' he says. 'It also boosts the immune system, suppresses bacteria and viruses that may be implicated in causing or aggravating the growth of cancer and stimulates white blood cells to mop up dead cancerous tissue and fight infection.'

Dr Wendy Denning treats many cancer patients who are having vitamin C therapy alongside conventional treatments and in her experience they work well together: 'The patients who do have vitamin C and minerals in between their doses of chemotherapy do much better in terms of maintaining their immune system, feeling better and being ready for the next round of chemo,' she says. Dr Denning does, however, urge patients to space their appointments out: 'I generally recommend leaving it for at least seventy-two hours after the chemotherapy and also avoiding having it two days before the chemotherapy,' she says. 'The last thing a patient wants when they are feeling nauseous from the chemotherapy is to be hooked up to another intravenous drip or for the chemotherapy to not do exactly what it is designed to do.' Dr Denning often adds magnesium and B vitamins into the solution too: 'I find that often cancer patients are deficient in these nutrients – particularly after chemotherapy or radiotherapy,' she says.

Beating End-stage Cancer

So how well does vitamin C work on its own – that is, without radiation or chemotherapy? Bryan Hubbard, co-publisher of *What Doctor's Don't Tell You* (a UK magazine he produces alongside his wife and best-selling author Lynne McTaggart), witnessed its miraculous effects first-hand. 'At the age of seventy-eight my mother Edie was diagnosed with end-stage breast cancer. The family doctor said he had never seen a case of breast cancer like it – her breast was just an open red sore – and he gave her three months to live. But I knew there were other options. Within a week we had booked an appointment with a qualified doctor who was pioneering alternative cancer therapies. He immediately put my mother on a drip, which was delivering very high levels of vitamin C and hydrogen peroxide. He also insisted on a radical change of diet. Six months later the family doctor bumped into my mother in the street and genuinely thought he'd seen a ghost. He could not believe his eyes and, like most people who cannot believe the evidence in front of them, he insisted on tests. My mother subjected herself to a mammogram that revealed that, indeed, the breast was completely free of cancer.'

And the name of that pioneering doctor? Dr Patrick Kingsley. For years Kingsley, who is now retired, treated thousands of patients at his clinic in the UK in Leicestershire. Those with end-stage cancer would travel miles to see him and in thousands of cases he turned patients' lives around. He has written about his experiences in his autobiography, *The Medical Detective – Memoirs of a Most Unusual Doctor*. 'I let people know before they came to see me that there was a distinct possibility, if they had cancer, that I would offer them intravenous vitamins and minerals, with vitamin C being the most important,' he says. 'I always started with 5 grams, just to make sure they felt better and I would give them a whole mix of B vitamins and minerals together with that. No end of times people rang me up afterwards and said, "Oh that was wonderful, I really felt so much better". Just about everybody who came to see me was in a nutritionally poor state.'

How Does IVC Work?

The fact that intravenous vitamin C can be toxic to tumours is now well established in the scientific literature,[20] although the exact mechanism by which it dissolves cancer is still being debated. What we do know is that at very high concentrations, vitamin C undergoes a transformation.

'After a certain level, around 50,000mg, vitamin C converts into a pro-oxidant and encourages cells in the body to produce hydrogen peroxide,' says Kingsley. Healthy white blood cells are able to make and break down their own peroxide to kill germs and fight foreign invaders. But cancer cells, lacking an essential enzyme, are not able to break down peroxide. It is therefore toxic to them.

Critics of vitamin C therapy will often cite a study by the Mayo Clinic as evidence that vitamin C therapy doesn't work. Shortly after Pauling and Cameron released the results from their ground-breaking vitamin C study, researchers from the Mayo Clinic ran a similar trial, but with one key difference: while Pauling and Cameron administered 10g vitamin C intravenously, the Mayo participants were given the same dose *orally*. The Mayo Clinic found that the vitamin C made no difference to survival rates, with the result that vitamin C therapy was dismissed as quackery.

But controversy surrounding the aforementioned study has now, finally, been put to rest. In 2004, scientists at the US National Institutes of Health found that blood concentrations of vitamin C when given intravenously were 6.6 times greater than when the same amount was given orally.[21] The authors of the study, both from conventional medical backgrounds, concluded that: 'The efficacy of vitamin C treatment cannot be judged from clinical trials that use only oral dosing.' As Professor Brighthope explains, 'You cannot achieve the extremely high physiological level that severely ill patients require by taking it orally.'

For deadly viruses, vitamin C injections can literally be a life-saver. During a polio epidemic in 1948–9 a virtually unknown practitioner from Pennsylvania, Dr Frederick Robert Klenner, cured every polio case he saw by using vitamin C injections,[22] and many doctors have been using vitamin C injections to treat viruses ever since: 'I use it a lot for people who have acute viral illness,' says Dr Wendy Denning. 'They will come into my office and say, "I feel dreadful, what can you do for me?" and I'll say, "I'm going to send you next door to the nurse and you're going to get a vitamin injection."'

The almighty anti-viral ability of vitamin C was once again brought to the fore in 2009. This time the world was watching. When news broke of a New Zealand dairy farmer who 'came back from the dead' thanks to high-dose vitamin C the story literally 'went viral'. After Alan Smith suffered an acute case of swine flu, the doctors wanted to turn off his life support, but his family demanded the hospital try intravenous vitamin C. The dairy farmer made a full recovery.[23] But it's not easy convincing nursing staff to administer vitamin C, as one of my readers from Queensland discovered. He recently left this comment on my blog: 'I was in a major hospital, diagnosed with swine flu; I had ampules of high doses of vitamin C [and] asked that they be put into my IV. Not only did they refuse, they confiscated my own property; they refused to give it back.'

Need to Know

'Before you give mega doses of vitamin C you must check for glucose-6-phosphate dehydrogenase (G6PD) deficiency,' says Dr Denning. 'If you give G6PD deficient patients high-dose vitamin C, it can cause damage of the red blood cells, and that can precipitate a fatal reaction. To this day, although I've checked every patient I've given high-dose vitamin C to, I've never yet seen a patient with that deficiency. But you can never be too careful.' Among the thousands of patients Patrick Kingsley tested, he only met two who had G6PD deficiency. 'I recommended intravenous hydrogen peroxide to them instead,' he says (see Chapter 9).

So how often should patients have vitamin C therapy? 'I would give it as often as the patient could manage – I would give it every day, if that was possible, but the vast majority of my patients came from such a long distance that I rarely gave it that often – usually it was twice a week. But I made sure they took large oral doses of vitamin C in between appointments.'

The Best Vitamin C Supplement

Liposomal (or lypo-spheric) vitamin C is great for those who can't afford vitamin C injections or for those on the road. Patrick Holford explains liposomal technology: 'It means that the vitamin C is encased in a 'liposome', which is a tiny bubble made out of the same material as a cell membrane,' he says. 'This "capsule" can be filled and used to deliver drugs for cancer and other diseases. In this way, the drug – or vitamin C in this case – is able to get directly into the cell itself to do its job.' Snip the sachet, mix in juice and take on an empty stomach.

So how do you know whether you're getting enough for optimal health? Dr Garry Gordon recommends regularly checking your vitamin C levels with urine test strips called VitaChek-C (available online). 'At roughly 25 cents each, these convenient indicators show the amount of vitamin C being metabolised and accordingly, circulating through the body,' says Dr Gordon. 'By looking at the colour change – matching against the colour chart – you can see if vitamin C levels are sufficient. The brighter the colour, the more vitamin C – so it's important to keep the strip bright to enable your body to work at the optimum level.'

Another product favoured by leading cancer specialists around the world (including Patrick Kingsley and Marcus Freudenmann) is Bio En'R-G'y C. 'It is an extremely good form of vitamin C. I used to find that even one gram of ordinary vitamin C gave me bowel problems, but I can take 4–6 grams of this powder in one go,' says Kingsley.

Once Kingsley got the patient's cancer 'under control', which often took him a matter of months, he would taper the treatment off 'or stop it completely'.

So how long does an IVC session last? 'You need to infuse it at a certain rate to achieve the right level of vitamin C in the blood,' explains Dr Denning. 'So 100 grams is generally given over one and a half to two hours and 50 grams is ideally given over one hour.'

It might sound tedious being tied up to a drip for that long, but for mum there were hidden benefits. 'It's like group therapy,' she announced when she walked in the door following her first session. During the hour and a half that it took for the vitamin solution to infuse, she'd made friends and swapped stories about everything from hydrogen peroxide and infrared saunas to dairy-free recipes and coffee enemas. 'Nothing is off-limits in that room,' mum said, eyes twinkling. When faced with the fear of losing your life, it seems people can lose their inhibitions too.

Others have reported similar bonding experiences from healing centres around the world. One reader took her mother to a clinic in the Bahamas when conventional US doctors had given up hope: 'A lot of the patients stick around in the meeting room/ waiting room to visit, and share stories and catch up. There are forty people all talking and laughing, talking about cancer and life. The returning patients talk about how bad their cancer was four, eight, ten, eighteen even twenty-eight years ago when they started coming to the clinic [and how] the cancer has since disappeared.'

Does IVC Work For Everyone?

No, is the short answer. 'I do have one patient with metastatic breast cancer who came to me recently and it did not work for her,' says Dr Denning. 'She's now trying something else her doctor is prescribing. But for the large majority of patients it's hugely beneficial.'

When someone with cancer isn't doing chemotherapy or radiotherapy, Dr Denning always recommends that they get their blood analysed by a laboratory in Greece. 'The lab is at the fore-front of molecular oncology and they will test against thirty to thirty-five alternative treatments and highlight what works best for a patient [see Chapter 10]. But what's been interesting for me, is that vitamin C has come up as being beneficial for almost every patient I've tested on so far, and that's not true of any other treatment.'

If your internal environment isn't properly prepared, how-ever, vitamin C won't work, according to Marcus Freudenmann, producer of the hit documentary *CANCER is Curable NOW*. 'Do you know that a lot of people go for high-dose vitamin C treat-ments and it doesn't work, it doesn't help, it doesn't do anything ... if they don't have high oxygen intake? Your body doesn't produce any hydrogen peroxide if there isn't enough oxygen to work alongside the high-dose vitamin C.' Mum always had ozone therapy alongside IVC, but Freudenmann's next piece of advice was new to her: 'When you go to clinics in Mexico and America they prime patients with vitamin K [found in green veg-etables] before they feed them vitamin C. It's an important co-factor.'[24]

Enzymes – the New Antioxidants?

In a 2008 paper entitled 'Enzymes and Cancer: A Look Toward the Past as We Move Forward',[25] integrative oncol-ogy expert Dr Keith Block writes about meeting a German doctor at a cancer conference at the National Institutes of Health: 'I asked him what the most exciting thing in cancer

▶

CAM (complementary and alternative medicine) in Europe was at that time. "Enzymes," he said. A bit surprised by his instantaneous response, I asked him what the second most exciting thing was. Again, with no hesitation he blurted out, "More enzymes!"'

The anonymous German doctor is not the only one to be evangelical about enzymes. Many leading cancer specialists, including Dr Leonard Coldwell, Dr Nicholas Gonzalez and Dr Garry Gordon, are similarly enthusiastic.

'Enzymes help to keep the blood less like ketchup and more like red wine,' says Dr Garry Gordon. Why might this be a bonus for cancer patients? 'Thick blood moves cancer more easily from one area to another,' Gordon explains. 'So you can't eliminate cancer without eliminating the thickness of blood.' Dr Gordon puts every cancer patient on an enzyme programme – generally Wobenzym (which is, interestingly, the second most popular pain therapy in Germany, outsold only by aspirin[26]).

Dr Leonard Coldwell refers to enzymes as the 'mailmen' of the body: 'They convert information into our biochemical system,' he says. Coldwell doesn't endorse enzyme supplements, however. Rather, he is a 'friend of juicing': 'All our food is cooked, preserved and pasteurised, meaning it is devoid of enzymes,' he says. 'So I tell everyone to invest in a juicer and juice organic vegetables. As a general rule you cannot mix vegetables with fruits, as the enzymes kill each other. The only exception to that rule is apples because of a specific form of enzymes they have.' Dr Coldwell recommends a combination of celery, carrot and apple juice every morning on an empty stomach as a way of boosting enzyme levels and detoxing the body.

▶

Leading cancer specialist Dr Nicholas Gonzalez has had great success treating patients with enzymes, coffee enemas (see Chapter 5) and individualized diets. 'For cancer patients we use large doses of orally ingested pancreatic enzymes,' he says. 'The average patient takes about 90 to 120 capsules of enzymes a day. They are spread throughout the day, six or seven doses, away from meals.'

It might sound monotonous, but according to Gonzalez, patients soon adapt: 'There is one patient in particular I'm thinking about who came to me in his forties. At the beginning he was constantly saying: "When are you going to reduce the enzymes?" Three or four years later all his liver tumours were gone, he was feeling great and I said, "Well, it's time to reduce the enzymes," and he said, "Are you sure you want to do that?" He's still on a full enzyme programme and that's eleven years later now. Most patients realise that it's not that tough to take pills when you're facing a deadly disease,' says Gonzalez. 'I have patients now in their mid-nineties that have been with me for twenty years; as long as they follow the diet and take their enzymes they're fine.'

Enzymes have been the key to survival for patients with a wide variety of cancers, including metastatic breast cancer, kidney cancer and leukaemia.[27] In one study where 107 women had undergone mastectomies for breast cancer, 84 per cent of those on enzymes (Wobenzym) survived more than five years, compared to 43 per cent on conventional therapy.[28] Another study of lung cancer patients suggested that enzymes reduced chemotherapy side effects and improved quality of life.[29] Dr Gonzalez

▶

explains: 'Enzymes selectively concentrate around the cancer cells and chew up the cell membranes and the cancer cell basically explodes.'

Before her diagnosis mum knew very little about enzymes; but she was quick to school up on this essential ingredient for good health. Every day she makes herself a tall glass of vegetable juice; she also takes Plantazyme, Rutozym (containing the enzyme Nattokinase), Bromelain (from pineapple) and Wobenzym.

Mum's programme was carefully put together with the help of a qualified health practitioner; be sure to always get the best advice on what's right for you.

A Cheap Shot

Ralph Moss, medical writer and cancer coach explains why we haven't heard more about vitamin C: 'No non-toxic, readily available agent has ever been approved by the Food and Drug Administration for the treatment of cancer. Vitamin C at retail sells for around five cents per gram. The cost of even 100 grams prepared for intravenous use is still very inexpensive compared to patented chemotherapy. I therefore don't think you will find many drug companies lining up to test and market such a readily available agent. And so the question of what vitamin C can do for patients – so fascinating and promising – has remained in limbo.'[30]

While recent research, released from the heart of the mainstream medical fraternity,[31] will go some way to silencing the 'quack-busters', it's unlikely to transform attitudes overnight: 'Oncologists will do what politicians do, and that is spin a story to suit a position that they've adopted. And the position that they have adopted is basically, "I make a diagnosis of cancer; I will treat the cancer with chemotherapy, radiotherapy or surgery – and there's nothing else that will help this patient,"' says Professor Brighthope.

But change is afoot. In Australia, doctors can now train in nutritional and environmental medicine and receive a fellowship or diploma and get CPD (continuing professional development) points for it. 'There will always be resistance, even hostility from the nutritional "flat-Earthers" – those who believe that "If you eat a balanced diet, then you cannot be deficient in essential nutrients" despite overwhelming evidence to the contrary,'[32] Professor Brighthope continues. 'But I believe the system will eventually change in line with the accumulating evidence, and research in the field of nutritional medicine is growing at a phenomenal rate,' he says. The number of practitioners who now offer IVC in the UK is testament to its growing popularity.

It's hard to put the nail in the coffin of something that's evidently helping to keep patients alive. Of course vitamin C is not the whole story in terms of cancer recovery – no one thing is. But nature has provided a magic tonic and many patients have felt blessed to find it.

●

CHAPTER 5

How Do You Take Your Coffee?

*'In pre-revolutionary France, a daily enema
after dinner was de rigueur.'*
Ralph Moss, medical writer and researcher

I f you ever find yourself on Portobello Road in London, take a moment to duck into Coffee Plant. There you will discover a mixture of local celebrities, clued-up tourists and coffee snobs all peering at the board and shouting out orders for 'long, skinny macs' and 'soya lattes' over the buzz of the latest Ibiza compilation. Coffee Plant has been keeping the Notting Hill set fuelled for over fifteen years with their organic, fairtrade beans and village vibe. It's the meeting place of choice for media types – the owner was once a journalist himself – and is regularly listed in the top five coffee shops in the UK.

But what few people know about this iconic establishment is that among the exotic roasts on the menu – the 'Old Brown Java', 'Rwandan Blend' and 'Strong French' – there is a curious entry called 'Gerson Blend'. And while wine-style tasting notes accompany the rest of the range, under this particular entry there is scant detail. The dispassionate description reads as follows: 'This is a specialist coffee for medical use only. It is always organic and always ground medium fine in one-kilogram packs.'

What could it possibly be used for, you might well wonder. A formula for chronic fatigue? A special blend for acute apathy? A prescription-only brew for jet-lag? For the uninitiated, 'Gerson Blend' could mean anything. But for those in the know, it means only one thing: coffee enemas – made famous by the German physician Max Gerson (see box page 85).

From Pharaohs to French Kings

Enemas are nothing new. In fact, they're as old as time. According to medical writer and researcher Ralph Moss, enemas are even mentioned in the Egyptian Ebers Papyrus (1500 BC): 'Millennia before, the Pharaoh had a "guardian of the anus", a special doctor one of whose purposes was to administer the royal enema.'

A daily coffee enema became a regular afternoon ritual for mum pretty soon after she was diagnosed with cancer. The process involves filling a hot-water-bottle-like contraption with tepid caffeinated coffee, hanging it from a bathroom towel rack and releasing the solution into the colon. The name of the game is to stimulate the liver.

'The coffee enemas are a simple technique that helps the liver work more efficiently,' says leading cancer specialist Dr Nicholas Gonzalez. 'They help the body neutralise, mobilise and excrete all the toxic debris that overloads the liver – including the metabolic toxins from the dead tumour.'

The Coffee Enema King

A few weeks after mum's diagnosis I had the privilege of interviewing Dr Jonathan Wright, a luminary in the alternative health world. When I asked him about mum's cancer, he replied: 'If she were my mum, I would send her to New York City to Nicholas Gonzalez right away. His track record is better than anyone's in the United States for helping people to get over their cancers.'

Dr Nicholas Gonzalez has been prescribing daily coffee enemas for his patients – along with individualised diets, enzymes and targeted supplements – for the last twenty-five years. One of his patients is a twenty-four-year survivor of metastatic breast cancer. 'I know of no other patient with stage-4 inflammatory breast cancer, that failed chemo, alive twenty-four years later,' says Dr Gonzalez.

The highly sought-after physician has had phenomenal success with a wide variety of cancers, including pancreatic cancer, considered by many to be the most deadly kind. The average survival time for advanced pancreatic cancer is just three months,[1] but for those under the care of Gonzalez, the outlook is different. One patient came to him in 1991 with stage-4 pancreatic cancer; he was riddled with tumours in his liver, lung, bones and both adrenal glands. His oncologist had given him two months to live and refused to treat him, saying, 'We're not going to make you miserable.' With nothing to lose, the man travelled to New York and started the Gonzalez programme, including the infamous daily enemas. The result? He lived for fourteen years. He died, at the age of eighty-five, following a car accident.

A pilot study led by Gonzalez and published in the peer-reviewed journal *Nutrition and Cancer*[2] in 1999 documented the most positive results for pancreatic cancer in the history of medicine. Out of eleven subjects with the disease, nine (81 per cent) lived for at least one year. Five of those nine survived for two years and four survived three years. In 1999 the remaining two patients were reported to still be 'alive and doing well'. To give you some idea of the monumental significance of these results, compare this study of Gonzalez's therapy with a trial of the chemotherapy drug Gemcitabine, published around the same time. Out of the 126 patients in this trial – more than ten times the number in Gonzalez's trial – not a single patient lived more than nineteen months.

Gerson Therapy

Dr Max Gerson developed the Gerson Therapy in the 1930s, initially as a cure for his own migraines, and eventually as a treatment for degenerative diseases such as cancer and diabetes. It is a nutrition-based programme that reawakens the body's power to heal itself. Gerson believed that tumours formed when the liver, pancreas and other organs were out of balance, so he prescribed daily juices, vitamin injections and coffee enemas to restore the body's natural equilibrium.

Patients on the Gerson Therapy typically consume about 6.8–9 kilograms of organically grown fruits and vegetables every day – mostly in the form of fresh juices. As you can imagine, that's a lot of grocery shopping. But for many people the relentless regime is worth the effort.

Dr Gerson claimed to have had a 50 per cent success rate[3] – nothing short of exceptional when you consider that 90–95 per cent of the patients he treated were considered terminal. Those suffering from melanoma seem to do particularly well on the diet. One study, published in a peer-reviewed journal,[4] compares the survival rates of melanoma patients being treated Gerson style, versus those having conventional treatment. Of 17 with stage-3 melanoma, 82 per cent of those on the Gerson diet were alive at five years, in contrast to 39 per cent of those undergoing conventional treatment.

Today the Gerson Institute is run by the tenacious Charlotte Gerson, Max's ninety-year-old daughter. She has dedicated her life to educating millions of people about the benefits of this non-toxic therapy and, despite her age, she is still touring the globe. Every year thousands of

▶

cancer patients emerge from the clinics – in Mexico and Hungary – cancer-free, and thousands more are getting well thanks to the legion of Gerson-trained practitioners worldwide. Kathryn Alexander is one of them. Her book, *Nutritional Healing: a Patient Management Handbook* is described by Charlotte Gerson as the 'bible' of the nutritional healer of the future.

Alexander has witnessed first-hand many cancer patients recover on the Gerson Therapy: 'I've currently got two patients who are cured of lymphoma. One lady had an abdominal tumour of thirteen centimetres by eight centimetres. She was on the therapy for eight months and when she went back to have another scan it was less than two centimetres.'

The aim of the Gerson Therapy is to rebuild the body at a cellular level: 'Gerson Therapy raises the energy capacity of cells through stimulating the mitochondria,' says Alexander. 'That's why the Gerson Therapy may not work for leukaemia patients. Because with leukaemia the white blood cells (neutrophils) don't have mitochondria that participate in energy production.'

Nurse's Little Helper

Book into any holistic health retreat today and you're likely to find colonics or enemas on the itinerary. But it might surprise you to know that enemas are actually as conventional as they come. 'Every hospital was once equipped with colon hydrotherapy machines or enemas,' says Matt Monarch a US-based raw-food guru. 'They were pretty much the first measure any nurse or doctor ever utilised when helping someone heal.' Ten years ago when Monarch left the corporate world in search of fulfilment, he found it through a clean-living lifestyle. He ditched the Standard American Diet (SAD) and became 100 per cent vegan, and today he travels the world with his wife, Angela Stokes-Monarch, and baby Oria, espousing the benefits of a raw-food diet and colon cleansing. His hugely popular *Raw Food World* TV show has reached audiences all over the world.

While some might dismiss coffee enemas as a hippy fad, they were actually included in the Merck Manual – considered the conventional medical Bible – right up until 1977. 'When I spoke to the editor, he said the only reason they took them out was because they thought it was a little "folksy",' says Gonzalez. 'They wanted to put more high-tech stuff in.'

Although coffee enemas might be written off as quackery, conventional medical literature is littered with research supporting their benefits. For over a century, coffee enemas have been used to treat a wide range of illnesses, from migraines and eczema to septic shock and psychological disorders. 'I have a paper from 1922, published in the *New England Journal of Medicine*, which describes how a group at Harvard Medical School successfully treated what we call today "bipolar", with enemas,' says Gonzalez. 'They got them off drugs and out of the hospital.'

Simple Solution

Talk of coffee enemas inevitably leads to questions such as, 'Is it hard to do?' and 'Does it hurt?' The answer to both questions is an emphatic 'No'. 'It is not hard to put a soft rubber tube in the rectum and let a pint of coffee in,' says Gonzalez. 'I've been doing it for over thirty-one years.'

In 1983 Gonzalez graduated from Cornell University with a medical degree. Back then, he had little knowledge of – or interest in – nutrition. During a post-graduate fellowship, however, Gonzalez completed a research study evaluating an aggressive nutritional therapy for advanced cancer. The highly controversial therapy was the brainchild of Dr William Donald Kelley, a country orthodontist who cured himself of pancreatic cancer through a 'trial-and-error' process. Gonzalez explains: 'I grew up on junk food, I used to eat chocolate for lunch in college ... Of course, then I met Kelley, and it changed my life.' Kelley fortuitously put together the therapy that saved his own life and the lives of countless others. One of the central tenets of this groundbreaking regime was coffee enemas.

How Mum Takes Her Coffee

- Pour four cups of filtered water into the coffee machine and add four tablespoons of organic coffee. Do not use a paper filter as they are filled with chemicals. (Dr Lloyd Jenkins from the Budwig Centre suggests using a nylon or metal permanent filter, or using a coffee machine that requires no filters.) A cafetiere is also fine to use.

- Allow the coffee to cool to body temperature. If mum forgets to make the coffee earlier, she'll put some ice cubes (made from filtered water) in the cup to cool it down.

- Take the tepid coffee to the bathroom and roll out a yoga mat. Cover it with an old towel (one that you don't mind staining). You also might like to have a pillow for your head and something to read or watch.

- Before filling the enema bag with coffee, ensure that

▶

you have completely locked the pinch clamp to block the flow of liquid.

- Fill the bag with coffee and hang it from a doorknob or towel rail – approximately 1 metre from the floor.

- Lubricate the catheter and your back passage – organic coconut oil is a good choice.

- Choose your position, get comfortable and insert the colon tube, so that it is about 25cm in.

- Turn the liquid flow on (by opening the pinch clamp) and let the water flow into your colon. If at any time you feel the urge to let it all out, first stop the liquid flow by pinching the clamp fully.

- Try and keep the coffee in for at least ten minutes and then release it down the toilet.

- Wash the enema kit with warm, soapy water and mild disinfectant, followed by a rinse with hot running water. In addition, you should periodically rinse the colon tube with hydrogen peroxide.

(Approved by Dr Nicholas Gonzalez.)

The New Sleeping Pill?

Prior to meeting Kelley, Gonzalez didn't touch coffee. 'I have an amphetamine-like reaction to coffee and never drink it,' says Gonzalez. 'If I have one cup I won't sleep for twenty-four to thirty-six hours. But the first time I did a coffee enema? I fell asleep.'

The soporific effect of coffee enemas is well known. Although mum has never fallen asleep at the wheel, so to speak, she finds the activity very relaxing. At around 4pm, most days, she rolls out the yoga mat, plumps a pillow and reads a book – or listens to an inspirational speaker – for fifteen to thirty minutes while the caffeine does its work. As someone who has a hard time letting go, she finds the ritual the perfect way to unwind. It gives her permission to stop everything and retreat to the bathroom, the one place guaranteed to be free of interruptions.

'Most patients report feeling relaxed when they do the coffee enemas,' says Gonzalez. So why does the morning latte make us buzz? 'Drinking coffee stimulates the sympathetic nervous system and shuts down the liver,' explains Gonzalez. When the sympathetic system switches on, the body prepares itself for 'fight or flight' and digestion and detoxification are put on hold. When you take coffee rectally, however, the opposite phenomenon occurs: 'It stimulates the parasympathetic nerves in the lower pelvis,' says Gonzalez. 'When these nerves are turned on, they feed back through a reflex to the liver, and within seconds the liver starts working more efficiently.' So while a double espresso might keep *you* wired for hours, a coffee enema will only liven up your liver.

But the benefits don't stop there. The coffee enema will also cleanse the blood, reduce inflammation and increase levels of glutathione, according to Kathryn Alexander. British-born Alexander completed her Gerson training in the USA, and over the last fifteen years she has lectured widely in the UK, USA and Europe. Now based on the Sunshine Coast, Australia, there is nothing she doesn't know about coffee enemas: 'Substances in the coffee, palmitates, activate the enzyme system glutathione-S-transferase seven-fold,' she says.

Glutathione (pronounced gloota-thigh-own) is a heavyweight when it comes to kicking cancer. According to Patrick Holford, British nutritionist and author of *Say No To Cancer*, glutathione 'deserves attention as it is perhaps the most important antioxidant within cells and has proven to be highly cancer-protective.' Glutathione has been shown to stimulate apoptosis[5] of malignant cells while leaving healthy cells unaffected. In other words, the antioxidant alerts the cancer cells that they've been living beyond their use-by date and it's time to die. Other studies have shown glutathione can reverse the development of neuroblastoma, cervical carcinoma and leukaemia[6] (see box below).

Glutathione – An Anti-cancer Hero

Glutathione is, according to a variety of leading health experts, 'the mother of all antioxidants',[7] like wearing a 'bullet-proof vest'[8] and an 'all-round cancer protecting agent'.[9]

Glutathione is rarely talked about in the mainstream health media, yet there are more than 89,000 medical articles about this multi-tasking molecule.[10] Not only does glutathione neutralise free radicals, it also boosts natural killer cells, controls inflammation and detoxifies the liver.

'It's the most important molecule you need to stay healthy and prevent disease,' enthuses *New York Times* best-selling author Dr Mark Hyman. 'It's the secret to prevent ageing, cancer, heart disease, dementia and more, and necessary to treat everything from autism to Alzheimer's disease.' Dr Hyman, who has been treating chronically ill patients for more than ten years, discovered that glutathione deficiency was a common denominator.

Glutathione operates in the liver – where it seizes toxins and ushers them out of the body. However, modern life is putting our natural healing capabilities to the test. 'There are a lot of things that reduce glutathione levels in the modern world, ranging from food toxins and environmental toxins

▶

to chronic illness and stress, so virtually all of us are subject to glutathione depletion,' says Chris Kresser, integrative practitioner and popular blogger. As we age our levels of glutathione start to decline, usually around the age of forty-five. These levels can dip by as much as 50 per cent.

So what can you do about it? Boosting your intake of foods rich in cysteine can help, since this amino acid plays a vital role in the production of glutathione. Eggs, meat, nuts, sweet potatoes, garlic and onions are all good sources. Or you could try supplementing with N-acetyl cysteine (NAC): 'If you can get NAC to cells, the cells will synthesise glutathione,' says Patrick Holford. Exercise can also increase your glutathione levels, along with milk thistle, selenium, B6 and B12 according to Dr Hyman.[11] If you're considering supplementing with glutathione itself, there are a few important rules to follow: 'Supplementing glutathione on its own is only mildly effective, since the fragile nutrient has a hard time surviving in the digestive tract,' says Holford. 'For that reason enteric-coated supplements are preferable, but another solution is to combine glutathione with anthocyanidins – antioxidants found in grapes, berries and beetroot. Anthocyanidins recycle glutathione, making it much more effective.'

Glutathione can also be administered intravenously, sublingually (under the tongue), nebulised and through enemas, according to Dr Mark Sircus, author and experienced physician. 'Adding glutathione to your treatment plan can boost your chances of survival by 20 per cent,' he says.

Back in Australia, mum is raising her glutathione levels

▶

in a number of ways. Along with daily coffee enemas, she is also taking a supplement called Cellgevity. It uses a specially patented technology to deliver cysteine to the cells, where it is transformed into glutathione. She has also started wearing special patches, said to increase levels of glutathione in the body by a whopping 454 per cent.[12]

Choose Your Position

There is a veritable karma sutra of possible coffee enema positions to choose from. Some people prefer to insert the catheter kneeling with their head to the ground – for yogis that's 'child pose' or 'rabbit pose' – while others like to administer the enema with one knee curled to the stomach. Others still decide to take it lying down. And while some experts believe the most effective way to stimulate the liver is by lying on the right side, others favour the left: 'I have seen grown people nearly come to blows over this question,' writes Ralph Moss. 'This is the CAM[13] equivalent of the war of the Big-Endians vs Little-Endians in Gulliver's Travels.'[14]

Ultimately, the choice is yours; but whichever way you choose to have your coffee, there are a few important rules that apply to everyone ...

Coffee Enema Dos and Don'ts

- Above all else, the coffee must be cooled to body temperature – the highly sensitive rectal area will not appreciate 'just off' the boil!

- The kind of coffee you use is also important: 'It has to be organic and medium roast,' advises Kathryn Alexander. Certain brands, such as S. A. Wilsons Gold Roast, have been specially blended with cancer patients in mind. 'Every single step in the production of our enema coffee and the operation of our facility has been certified to organic standards, right down to the products we use to clean the floors,' says the creator, Scott Wilson. Independent research shows that Wilsons coffee is up to 48 per cent higher in caffeine and up to 87 per cent higher in palmitic acid, providing a powerful boost to glutathione levels and anti-cancer enzymes. Despite being an American company S. A. Wilsons offers free shipping to Australia, New Zealand and Canada. Mum recently switched to the bespoke blend and reports that the beans have a pleasing 'peanutty' aroma. The aforementioned 'Gerson Blend' is, of course, a great option for those in the UK; you can simply phone up Coffee Plant and have it delivered to your door. 'It is sold in one-kilogram bags and this is the most cost-effective way I have found to buy coffee for the enemas,' says Vincent Crewe, a loyal customer and natural cancer survivor.

- Before you take the plunger, you will also need to purchase a slim PVC catheter or rubber colon tube to attach to the enema nozzle. This piece of apparatus does not usually come with the enema kit. When mum first did an online search for 'colon tube' she ended up on a porn site (don't ask). So to spare you the same ordeal, the website where mum eventually procured the 'small French' colon tube is included in the Resources.

- Next question: how far up does it need to go? 'Twelve to eighteen inches – or about twenty-five centimetres,' says Gonzalez (or the same length as a Subway roll, as my brother's girlfriend helpfully pointed out).

- The good news is, you don't have to keep replacing the tube, as Gonzalez explains: 'The colon tube will last twenty years, they don't break down, you just occasionally put some [35 per cent food-grade] hydrogen peroxide through it to sterilise it.'

Coffee Enemas Are Not For You If . . .

'Generally we don't recommend coffee enemas for pregnant women and they may be contraindicated in those who are suffering from bleeding of the bowel,' says Kathryn Alexander. 'We still give enemas to people even if they don't *have* a bowel; you can administer it through an irrigation kit.' Those who have had part of their colon removed should have no problem doing enemas the normal way, according to Alexander.

None of Kathryn Alexander's patients has ever reported negative side effects from coffee enemas: 'Not one, no infection, nothing,' she says. In the twenty-five years of prescribing coffee enemas, not one of Gonzalez's patients has reported complications either. To prove their safety, Gonzalez took eight 'strong' coffee enemas a day for a period of six weeks when he was a student. In *One Man Alone* Dr Gonzalez reports the experiment yielded 'no adverse effect and no change in my electrolytes'.

However, if you are feeling a little depleted post enema, then drinking an antioxidant-rich juice will replenish your electrolytes. Dr Lloyd Jenkins, a naturopathic doctor from the Budwig Centre in Germany, suggests drinking a freshly made carrot and apple juice or a glass of leafy green vegetable juice for every coffee enema.

A Double Asspresso?

Patients of Gonzalez are required to have four enemas a day: 'Two in the morning, back to back; two in the afternoon back to back,' he says. 'So two pints in the morning, holding each pint for ten minutes, and the same in the afternoon.' Those who are following the Gerson Therapy (see box, page 85) are expected to do five coffee enemas a day. 'The cancer patient is producing toxins from the tumour twenty-four seven,' says Kathryn Alexander. 'The cancer is polluting the circulation, the blood ... so doing a coffee enema at regular intervals keeps the circulation clean and the pathways of detoxification stimulated.'

If you're feeling adventurous, you might also like to try a wheatgrass enema. Clients staying at the luxurious Mullum Sari retreat in Byron Bay can choose to have either coffee or wheatgrass in their daily colonic. 'The wheatgrass enema is lesser known, but it offers so many benefits for cancer patients,' says retreat manager Vicki Standley. 'Wheatgrass is jam-packed with chlorophyll and that brings more oxygen to the body. When cells are deprived of oxygen that's when they start becoming cancerous [see Chapter 9].' According to Standley, doing a wheatgrass enema is more effective than downing a shot: 'That way it goes straight to your colon without going through your digestive system first and it hits your liver straight after that.' How to do it? Simply add a shot of wheatgrass (50ml) to your enema bag along with filtered water. Bottoms up!

What the People Say

When mum first heard about coffee enemas, she was already having ozone therapy and vitamin C injections, taking enzymes, supplements and hydrogen peroxide and addressing her emotional health through a variety of different therapies. For her, the coffee enema was one more weapon to add to her arsenal. And it seems her patchwork approach is not unusual.

Over the last two years, we have heard from many others who, like mum, have chosen to combine various alternative therapies. Vincent Crewe, for instance (who you will hear more from in Chapter 12), uses coffee enemas along with infrared saunas, ozone therapy, apricot kernels, enzymes and more. Six years on from a diagnosis of metastatic colon cancer (spread to his liver) Vincent is fighting fit.

'For the first two years I did one coffee enema every day without fail,' says Vincent. 'But now I only do it twice a week.' A salt-of-the-earth Yorkshire type, Vincent wasn't shy about sharing his coffee enema experiences: 'Obviously, you're clumsy with everything when you first start. I used to use an old bath towel, but I'm more sophisticated now: I use a baby's bath mat which is plastic, so you don't have to worry about spills.' Vincent urges those about to embark on a coffee enema regime to stick with it: 'When I first tried it I could only hold the coffee for about five seconds, but within a few sessions I built up to fifteen minutes.' Adding half a tablespoon of (aluminium-free) bicarbonate of soda to the enema can help you retain the solution, according to Vincent: 'You can put all sorts in the enema … black strap molasses can also help with retention.'

Coffee enemas have also been an essential part of the recovery regime for forty-three-year-old Nicola Corcoran, a breast cancer survivor. 'These days I use coffee enemas for pain relief – particularly headaches,' says Nicola. 'I also do them when I feel like I'm coming down with something – like a cold or a tummy bug. Green juices, infrared saunas [see Chapter 7] and coffee enemas usually stop anything from taking hold.'

Better than BOTOX?

Coffee enema converts report luminous skin, flatter stomachs and feelings of 'euphoria'[15] thanks to this so-called 'freaky' ritual. Even Simon Cowell relies on regular enemas to keep his eyes sparkling.[16] Claudette from Paris, a subscriber of my blog, started coffee enemas as a way to detox her liver, but quickly found there were other bonuses: 'For as long as I can remember I've had terrible rings under my eyes. But when I started doing coffee enemas? They vanished. An hour after doing an enema my dark rings completely disappear.' Some claim a quick 'coffee break' can stop a cold in its tracks, while others swear enemas are the ultimate hangover cure.

Nicola, Vincent and mum have much in common. After undergoing surgery to remove cancerous tumours, they all refused follow up with chemotherapy and radiotherapy. Instead they opted to supercharge their immune systems and detoxify their bodies with a raft of different treatments. Today, all three report feeling 'better than ever'.

While oncologists have been known to warn against coffee enemas, evidence suggests they can be enormously beneficial for patients undergoing conventional treatment. In 1990, researchers at an oncology department in Austria found that coffee enemas allowed patients to handle higher amounts of chemotherapy.[17] The researchers' recommendation was: 'If a pharmaceutical company could make a drug that would do what the coffee enema did, they could give higher doses of chemotherapy,' says Alexander. 'Because the coffee enema actually protects the liver from the oxidative damage from chemotherapy.'

Gotta Have Faith

If prospective patients are anxious about doing coffee enemas, Gonzalez gently urges them to go elsewhere: 'Sometimes people come to me because their cousin wants them to come or the health-food store owner sent them, but they don't believe in me or my programme,' says Gonzalez. 'I can see it in the first minute I'm sitting with them. They're in a state of anxiety. How are they going to get well in a state of anxiety?'

Nutrition and detoxification are just part of the key to recovery, according to Gonzalez. Belief in the possibility of healing is also critical: 'I've had patients that were so sick ... but they had such strong faith in what we did, we put them on the programme and they got well,' he says. 'When people believe in something it creates a sense of relaxation and that's when healing occurs.'

Gonzalez Therapy: Dispelling the Myths

Thanks to Dr Gonzalez's remarkable results, the National Cancer Institute (NCI) agreed to fund a large-scale clinical trial in 1998, pitching the cancer drug Gemcitabine (Gemzar) against Gonzalez's own protocol. Dr Gonzalez hoped the venture would help vindicate his treatment and kick-start an era of co-operation between conventional scientists and alternative researchers. But it wasn't to be. In his latest book, *What Went Wrong: the Truth Behind the Clinical Trial of the Enzyme Treatment of Cancer*, Gonzalez documents how the study was mismanaged, how he had no control over the selection of patients and how his therapy was thwarted in various ways that were subsequently confirmed by regulatory authorities. This book sets the record straight.

While working as a medical student with Dr Kelley, Dr Gonzalez noticed that his mentor would regularly take time to speak to patients about their lives: their hopes, their fears and their relationships. 'One day I asked Dr Kelley: "What percentage of cancer is nutritional/biochemical, what percentage is psychological and what percentage is spiritual?"' recalls Gonzalez. 'Kelley responded by saying: "It's 100 per cent nutritional/biochemical." Which is the answer I wanted. He waited ten seconds and then he said, "It's 100 per cent psychological." He then waited ten more seconds and said, "It's 100 per cent spiritual in every single human being, including you."'

Enemas: a Path to Enlightenment?

Checking into an ashram in India or following a shaman in Peru might be the more typical choice for those seeking a spiritual awakening. But according to Matt Monarch you can also reach nirvana on your bathroom floor. 'There are a lot of yogi gurus who say, "If you want to be a disciple of mine, you've got to cleanse the colon",' says Monarch. 'When there is less toxicity in your cells there's room for life and vibration.'

Coffee enemas can also balance mood, according to natural cancer survivor Nicola Corcoran: 'The most surprising benefit from the coffee enemas is how clear it leaves me emotionally,' she says. 'If I'm feeling a little emotionally toxic (anxious, envious, off-track) then I do one for clarity.'

Last Christmas mum presented me with a coffee enema kit – undoubtedly one of the more unusual stocking fillers I've ever received. For the last few months, I too have taken the plunge. Friends have since complimented me on my clear complexion and healthy glow, and when I've revealed my health secret reactions have ranged from blushes to hearty guffaws. A few friends have asked for more details; others just don't want to know.

But while some might find the whole concept distasteful, cancer patients would do well to consider the alternative: when chemotherapy is accidentally spilled in any medical centre, it's considered a major biohazard and a team wearing special outfits resembling space-suits is called in to swiftly clear up the toxic mess. And yet, somehow, flooding someone's body with these chemical agents is okay and doing a coffee enema is a dangerous deal? The mysteries of Ancient Egypt are nothing compared to modern medicine.

CHAPTER 6

•

Getting Clean

'If we were a food, we would not be safe to eat.'
Mark Hyman, *The Blood Sugar Solution*[1]

I often wonder what it would be like to travel back in time. Say 500 years. Maybe not to Elizabethan London, with the open sewage and plague-stricken streets, but further afield. I long to know what it would be like to taste an apple from a medieval orchard, to swim in a pristine lake and to breathe in pure, fresh air. I fantasise about taking great big gulps of it, filling my body with oxygen free from mercury, lead, pesticides, herbicides and the 80,000[2] or so other chemicals that have been released into our environment since 1900. What would it taste like? How would it make me feel? Would I become brainier and better looking? Would my skin glow and hair shine? Would I be able to run like the wind? Would cancer even exist?

It wasn't until the eighteenth century that the first reports of cancer appeared in scientific literature, according to Danica Collins, natural health journalist and editor of the *Underground Health Reporter*: 'Cancer of the scrotum was found in chimney sweeps in 1775, caused by soot particles and nasal cancer found in users of snuff in 1761.' While some ancient cases of cancer did exist, recent research suggests that it is largely a modern, man-made disease. After examining hundreds of Egyptian mummies, researchers from the University of Manchester found only one isolated case of the condition. Professor Rosalie David at the Faculty of Life Sciences at Manchester University said: 'In industrialised societies, cancer is second only to cardiovascular disease as a cause of death. But in ancient times, it was extremely rare. There is nothing in the natural environment that can cause cancer. So it has to be a man-made disease, down to pollution and changes to our diet and lifestyle.'[3]

Today, early cancers are so common that autopsy studies of middle-aged and older people have revealed that almost everyone's body contains them.[4] On average, one out of two men has prostate cancer, 39 per cent of women have tumours in their breasts[5] and virtually all people between the ages of fifty and seventy have small tumours in their thyroids. Bottom line? If we want to make cancer ancient history, we need to clean up our environment.

Too Big to Ignore

In America in 2010, the President's Cancer Panel issued a landmark report suggesting that public health officials have 'grossly underestimated' the extent of environmentally induced cancer among the 1.5 million Americans diagnosed with the disease annually.[6] Commenting on the finding, author and physician Dr Mark Sircus, who offers a unique, non-toxic and inexpensive protocol for cancer patients says: 'Oncologists and medical officials tend to make light of the threat from environmental hazards, as do all people who live in big cities that are heavily polluted.' Those who work in the field of holistic health, however, have long known that man-made chemicals are strongly linked to cancer, and that the key to recovery is getting them out. As Dr Rashid A. Buttar, renowned physician, detox expert and author of *The 9 Steps to Keep the Doctor Away*,[7] says: 'Until toxicity is effectively addressed, no significant advance in cancer survival will ever happen.'

Unfortunately, mainstream medicine has been slow on the uptake. 'We've been trying for years to engage with the UK medical community with, if I'm honest, only limited success,' says Jamie Page, founder and CEO of the British-based charity the Cancer Prevention and Education Society. 'There's nothing harder than trying to convince an intelligent person that they're wrong.' Defenders argue that there is not enough evidence linking chemicals to cancer but, for obvious ethical reasons, it's not possible to submit humans to randomised chemical trials.

For many years Jamie Page, who has a degree in chemistry, worked in the pharmaceutical industry. 'But I couldn't understand why we were putting all this effort, all this money, into developing cures for cancer when we weren't addressing chemicals as a possible cause. Anti-smoking campaigns have prevented many tobacco-related diseases. We think action on chemicals can bring similar benefits to public health.' According to Page, the two types of cancer that have been going up in the last thirty to forty years are cancers of the hormone system and cancers of the immune system: 'Things like non-Hodgkin's lymphoma,' says Page. 'And it's simple in my mind. The hormone system and immune system are at the front line of chemical exposure.'

What Our Future Holds

Our bodies have become toxic dumping grounds. Endocrine-disrupting chemicals, heavy metals and pesticides now course through our veins and no one – regardless of age, occupation or postcode – is clean. In 2005 the Environmental Working Group shocked the world with their groundbreaking study showing that even babies are loaded with harmful substances. Researchers analysed newborn babies and found 287 chemicals and other toxins – including fire retardants, DDT and heavy metals – in their blood. One hundred and eight of the chemicals they discovered are known carcinogens.[8]

'A baby born today has a thousand times more lead in their bones than 700 years ago,'[9] says Dr Garry Gordon, co-founder of the American College for Advancement in Medicine (ACAM). 'The mother uses the child's body as a wastebasket to get rid of her lead, mercury and other toxins.' Terrifying, when you consider that the level of lead in your blood is a strong predictor of life expectancy.[10] Even the breast milk of nursing Arctic women has been found to be dangerously high in PCBs and mercury[11] – in other words, these chemicals are now unavoidable and their effects impossible to ignore.

Thanks to the march of modern industry, modern medicine and industrialised farming we are being systematically poisoned every minute of every day: from the mobile phone alarm in the morning to the microwave dinner at night, from the bowl of carcinogenic cereal to the computer we never shut down ... the onslaught is endless and the research frightening.

'Bisphenol A [BPA], phthalates, perfluorochemicals, polychlorinated biphenyls – the names don't exactly roll off the tongue, but you don't have to be able to pronounce them to be hurt by them,' writes renegade American physician Dr William Campbell Douglass II, in a recent article in *The Douglass Report*. 'These and other chemicals are making you fat, sick, weak and maybe one day dead. They're turning men into ladies and boys into girls ... And in everyone, these toxic ingredients are just the recipe for cancer, heart disease, sexual dysfunction and more.'[12]

More than 130 studies have found evidence of BPA's detrimental effect on human health,[13] linking it to – among other things – breast, prostate and brain cancer.[14] Then there is the issue of pesticides (workers who spray fields with certain substances are twice as likely to contract melanoma) and our love affair with diagnostic radiation: give a child two or three CT scans and you triple their risk of developing brain cancer.[15] And as for heavy metals? Just turn on the tap to get your fix of lead and mercury. You'll find 643 studies linking mercury with cancer[16] on the website Toxline and that's just the tip of the dirty iceberg. 'You could make just as strong a case about lead or cadmium or even arsenic – the point is that these things are threatening the health of the entire world,' says Dr Gordon.

With a new chemical synthesised every twenty-seven seconds[17] it might seem futile to fight the relentless foreign invasion, but studies have repeatedly shown that just a few small changes can go a long way to reducing your toxic load: 'If we add up all of the things that cause cancer and begin to eliminate them one by one we can reduce cancer rates by large amounts,' reassures Dr Mark Sircus.

You don't need to do everything, but you *can* do something. In this chapter you will learn steps you can take to shore up your defences (with nature as a powerful ally) and minimise your exposure to carcinogens, whether you're at home, having a check-up or flying over the Atlantic.

In Your Home

Your home should provide a sanctuary from the polluted world outside, but many homes are, in fact, chemical cocoons. The US-based Environmental Protection Agency (EPA) has suggested there are far higher levels of toxins inside our homes than outside.[18] One hundred times more, to be precise.

So where do these chemicals come from? 'Formaldehydes are in cheap furniture like pressed woods, there are several very toxic chemicals in carpets and there are volatile organic compounds (VOCs) in paints,' says Frank D. Wiewel, founder of the grassroots organisation People Against Cancer.[19] Formerly a rock star,

Wiewel swapped recording studios for health research almost thirty years ago. In 1985 he was accompanying his sick father-in-law to an alternative cancer clinic when it was summarily shut down at the instigation of the National Cancer Institute. Wiewel has been a leading figure in the fight for health freedom ever since.

Carpets are one of the biggest culprits for at-home toxicity, but compact fluorescent light bulbs (CFLs) are close behind, according to Wiewel. 'These bulbs contain mercury,' he says. 'Originally there was supposed to be a toxic waste dump to dispose of them, but a facility was never established.' The upshot? 'The mercury now goes back into the environment: our water supplies, the air,[20] the food – one teaspoon of mercury can contaminate an acre of lake,' says Wiewel. 'Mercury causes the suppression of natural killer cells. These are the cells we have to use in our bodies to fight cancer.'

Mercury also displaces other key nutrients: 'There's no question in my mind that mercury squanders selenium, which is a very important antioxidant in the body,' says British cancer expert Dr Patrick Kingsley. 'It also depletes vitamin C.'

And what about the king of convenience – the ubiquitous microwave oven? 'It kills the enzymes and creates a monster food ... yet nobody talks about it,' says Burton Goldberg, cancer coach and alternative medicine expert. According to one of Germany's leading oncologists, Dr Ursula Jacob, areas in Japan that have more microwaves have more cancers.[21] And in Russia, microwave ovens were banned between the years 1976 and 1987.[22] 'Russian researchers found decreased nutritional value, cancer-making compounds and brain-damaging radiolytics in virtually all microwave-prepared foods,' explains Andreas Moritz, Ayurvedic practitioner and medical intuitive. 'Radiation from the microwave has also been found to accumulate in kitchen furniture, becoming a constant source of radiation in itself.' So even if the microwave languishes on the counter, waiting for your other half to heat up the leftover bolognese, you could still be suffering from its deleterious effects.

Non-stick pans are also a bad idea since they contain perfluorochemicals. 'PFCs have been linked to hypothyroidism, immune system disorders, reproductive problems, cancer and more ... You'll find various PFCs in anything wrinkle-free, stain-resistant, heat-proof and non-stick,'[23] writes Dr Campbell Douglass II.

It's safe to say chemicals have conquered every inch of our home. There's even the opportunity to absorb carcinogens on the loo: 'BPA is in recycled paper products – including toilet paper,' says Campbell Douglass. 'When you touch it the BPA can actually penetrate your skin.' That's right – BPA isn't just limited to the lining of tinned food, as you may have read in the news. In fact, according to Marcus Freudenmann, producer of the hit documentary *CANCER is curable NOW*, it's even leached from contact lenses. But before you rush to stock up on 'BPA-free' products, a word of caution: 'BPA-free products often contain a chemical called BPS and the two have a lot more in common than their first two letters,' says Campbell Douglass. 'They're both chemical hormones that mimic oestrogen in the human body, disrupting the endocrine system and setting you up for illness and disease.' Although BPS is slightly weaker than its chemical cousin, a new study found we absorb nineteen times more of the BPS than the BPA through our skin.[24] The answer? Whenever you can, opt for glass and steel, wear spectacles and wash your hands after touching receipts – they also contain these chemicals. As for toilet paper – you might have to roll with that for now.

Phthalates (pronounced THA-lates) are another class of chemicals that get around. You'll find these hormone disruptors in plastic toys (including sex toys), shower curtains, household air fresheners[25] and 'just about anything scented', according to Campbell Douglass. 'Phthalates have been linked to stupidity in girls and motor skills delays in boys,' he writes.[26] In 2012 a Swedish study revealed that children's bodies can absorb the phthalates found in PVC flooring.[27] And while the jury is still out on whether the chemicals cause cancer, there's been enough damning evidence for a number of countries, including Denmark, to ban them outright.[28]

Then there's formaldehyde. It's found in everything from cheap furniture and wallpaper to shopping bags and detergent. This chemical, famously used by the artist Damien Hirst to preserve his artwork, was recently classified as carcinogenic by the US Department of Health and Human Services.[29] Research by the Netherlands Cancer Institute found a strong link between high formaldehyde exposure in funeral-home workers and leukaemia.

But you don't have to be in the business of embalming to increase your toxic load – as I discovered the hard way. In 2012 a biofeedback session (see Chapter 11) revealed my body was high in formaldehyde. Why would that be? I wondered, drawing a blank. It was only as this book was going to press that I discovered the most likely cause – central heating. In 2011 I replaced all the radiators in my London apartment, which I now know can offgas large amounts of formaldehyde in the first year following installation. Some believe they account for the largest source of formaldehyde in the home. Had I known this before I would have bought some anti-formaldehyde radiator paint.[30]

What you can do

- **Try a new lick of paint** 'We look for paints that have low or no volatile organic compounds [VOCs],' says Frank Wiewel.

- **Avoid the new carpet smell** 'When I recently bought a carpet I asked the people at the warehouse to roll it out and let it offgas there for three months,' says Wiewel. 'I then brought it home, steam cleaned it – without any perfume or fragrance – and ventilated the room for weeks afterwards.'

- **Choose nude floors** Instead of carpeting you could opt for sustainable hardwood floors with small rugs made from natural fibres.

- **Use glass and steel** Switching to fresh organics and using glass and steel for storage have been shown to reduce BPA levels in urine by 60 per cent in three days, according to a US study in 2010.[31]

- **Ditch plastic wrap for Abeego** Made from hemp, cotton fabric, beeswax and tree-resin, this handy, natural cling film is better for the environment and for you.

- **Pan it** 'Trash the Teflon and break out Grandma's cast-iron skillets instead,' suggests Dr William Campbell Douglass II.[32]

- **Use pantry ingredients to clean** 'Bicarb neutralises odours, removes stains and can be left overnight to clean the oven,' says Janey Lee Grace, author of *Look Great Naturally ... Without Ditching the Lipstick*. Bicarb is also a cheap way to help keep cancer at bay (see Chapter 13).

- **Keep indoor plants** According to NASA scientists, one peace lily can remove pollutants like formaldehyde from the air around it.[33]

- **Buy beeswax, not fragranced, candles** 'Instead of polluting, they'll actually improve the quality of your air indoors by boosting negative ions,' says Lee Euler, author and publisher of the highly acclaimed newsletter *Cancer Defeated!*

- **Deal with pests naturally** Families of children who had developed leukaemia were about three times as likely to have employed the use of a professional exterminator in their home than those who did not have a child with cancer,[34] according to research from the University of California at Berkeley.

- **Work from (your newly naturalised) home a few days a week** You can only ask!

In Your Water

In our post-recession world, asking for 'just tap' has become du jour. But the unpalatable truth is that pesticides, heavy metals, hormones, drugs and even rocket fuel[35] regularly make their way into the water system. How do these contaminants get there?

- Pesticides and herbicides are drawn into the supply as rain washes over the land.

- Heavy metals are picked up from pipes and joint fixtures.

- Hormones such as oestrogen contaminate the water system, thanks largely to women on the contraceptive pill. Chris Woollams, founder of CANCERactive and author of *Oestrogen: the Killer in Our Midst,* says 'the female sex hormone is one of the major drivers of many cancers. Not just breast cancer, but endometrial, cervical, colon, testicular and prostate cancer, as well as brain tumours. One source of unwanted oestrogen is tap water in big cities where the water is recycled.'

So should you head for the hills? The grass might be greener in the countryside, but not necessarily the water: 'Generally speaking, farmers are healthier than the average person,' says

British nutritionist and author Patrick Holford. 'Yet there is a disproportionate increase in the incidence of several cancers, including leukaemia, non-Hodgkin's lymphoma and cancers of the brain and prostate.' Could agrochemicals be to blame? Roundup, the world's best-selling herbicide, has been correlated with a higher risk of multiple myeloma,[36] as well as endocrine disruption, birth defects[37] and DNA damage.[38] Despite previous safety claims, a recent report found that glyphosate, the chemical in Roundup, was in fact capable of entering the ground water supplies.[39] Over in China, studies have linked nitrates from fertilisers to stomach cancer.[40] In fact, in 2013 the Chinese government admitted to the existence of 'cancer villages', which it attributes to severe water and air pollution.

Then there are the chemicals that are *purposely* added to our water supplies. Since the late 1800s chlorine has been added to defend against harmful bacteria, but it could be contributing to the cancer epidemic. 'Chlorine is a very well-known cancer-causing agent,' says the widely respected naturopath and clinical nutritionist David J. Getoff. According to the US Council of Environmental Quality, 'Cancer risk among people drinking chlorinated water is 93 per cent higher than among those whose water does not contain chlorine.'[41] Breast cancer, which now affects one in every eight women in the UK, has recently been linked to chlorine. A study carried out in Hartford, Connecticut found that, 'Women with breast cancer have 50 per cent to 60 per cent higher levels of organochlorines (chlorination by-products) in their breast tissue than women without breast cancer.'[42] It's worth noting that not all countries think it's a good idea to pour bleach into their water. More than 2500 municipalities around the world purify their water supplies with ozone, including Los Angeles, Paris, Montreal, Moscow, Kiev, Singapore, Brussels, Florence, Turin, Marseilles, Manchester and Amsterdam, according to Nathaniel Altman, author of *The Oxygen Prescription: the Miracle of Oxidative Therapies*.[43] Interestingly, during the 1984 Olympic Games held in Los Angeles, the European teams insisted the swimming pools be treated with ozone (as opposed to chlorine) or they would not participate in events.[44]

What you can do

- **Buy a reverse osmosis (RO) filter** The system, which can be fitted underneath your kitchen sink, will remove approximately 95 per cent of all nasties, as well as filtering unpleasant tastes and odours. However, if you go down this route, it's important to remineralise your water. Naturopath Jo Coates from Perth, Western Australia says: 'Reverse osmosis water has no life energy, no minerals and reacts quickly with CO_2 to become very acidic.'

- **Install a shower filter** According to Dr Lance Wallace from the US Environmental Protection Agency: 'Showering is suspected as the primary cause of elevated levels of chloroform in nearly every home because of chlorine in the water.'[45] After discovering that chlorine levels in the water in Perth were particularly high,[46] mum decided she wasn't taking any chances; she took the drastic (and expensive) measure of installing a whole-house filter, which purifies the water as soon as it enters the house system.

- **Carry filtered water around in a stainless steel bottle** Plastic bottles leach phthalates and BPA. Added to that is the huge environmental cost of drinking water from plastic bottles ... and the fact that 40 per cent of bottled water actually *is t*ap water.[47]

- **Flush your body clean** 'Drinking plenty of purified water allows nutrients to flood your cells while pushing toxins out. The body is like a river; as long as the water is flowing, we really can dump a lot of stuff in there and it cleans itself,' says leading cancer specialist Dr Leonard Coldwell.

In Your Food

Did you know there might be radioactive substances in your fruit and vegetables? It was news to me; as someone who scours health journals daily and regularly commiserates with slow-food supporters I was shocked that I'd missed this one. But a quick Google search confirmed the worst: over forty countries now approve irradiation as a way of extending the shelf life of certain foods, including fruits, vegetables, poultry and red meat.[48] Thankfully, food-labelling regulations in the UK ensure that any irradiated foods or ingredients are identified with the words 'irradiated' or 'treated with ionising irradiation'.[49] So for now, it's possible to avoid chomping down on a radioactive carrot. Although it pained me to read recently that we might one day be seeing in supermarkets bread that will last for sixty days, thanks to 'sophisticated' microwave zapping.[50]

For those who still question the value of organic food – those who are content with the antibiotics and hormones, the use of herbicides and pesticides and the suffering of animals on industrial farms – ponder this: results from a £12 million, four-year EU study suggest that organic fruits and vegetables have up to 50 per cent higher levels of cancer-fighting antioxidants than their non-organic cousins. Salvestrols – plant chemicals capable of selectively killing cancer cells – are also found in greater amounts (see Chapter 13).

So while a shiny, perfectly formed fruit may look delicious, there may be poison in every bite. 'The average conventionally grown apple has twenty to thirty artificial chemicals on its skin, even after rinsing,' writes Joshua Rosenthal in his book *Integrative*

Nutrition. For Rosenthal, founder of the Institute for Integrative Nutrition in the US (the world's largest nutrition school), eating organic is the cornerstone of good health: 'Fresh organic produce contains more vitamins, minerals, enzymes and other micronutrients than intensively farmed produce,' he says. 'Pesticides, which are present in most commercial produce, must be processed by our immune systems and have been shown to cause cancer as well as liver, kidney and blood diseases.'

The rapid rise of genetically modified (GM) food is also cause for alarm. In America as many as 85 per cent of the processed foods on store shelves contain GM ingredients[51] (compared to only 5 per cent in Europe[52]). The new technology is hailed as the answer to world hunger, but the ubiquity of GM could have serious consequences. In 2012 a French study shocked the world when it showed that rats fed on GM maize for two years developed large mammary tumours and severe liver and kidney damage.[53] Commenting on the study, Dr Michael Antoniou, a molecular biologist from King's College London said: 'This research shows an extraordinary number of tumours developing earlier and more aggressively – particularly in female animals. I am shocked by the extreme negative health impacts.'[54] While it's beyond the scope of this book to delve deeper into the GM rabbit hole, I'd encourage anyone who is interested to check out Jeffrey Smith's groundbreaking documentary *Genetic Roulette*.

Lead in Your Cereal?

On the box you see a sun-kissed wheat field and a 'heart healthy' tick, but your morning cereal is not the nutritious food you think it is. According to research it could be full of battery toxins and other heavy metals: 'With some

▶

cereals, you can take a magnet and put it underneath the bowl and move it around because there is so much lead in it,' says Marcus Freudenmann. So how does lead – which is extremely neurotoxic and cytotoxic[55] – make its way into your breakfast? 'It comes from the fortified iron they add in,' explains Freudenmann. 'Companies often don't use a pure form of iron and German studies have found it is often contaminated with lead, nickel and cadmium.' As if that wasn't bad enough, studies from Switzerland and Germany have found that cereal boxes might also be leaching carcinogenic chemicals into your morning flakes.[56] The harmful substances, which are said to cause inflammation of the internal organs, appear to come from the recycled paper that cereal boxes are made from.

Shake up your breakfast

Swap cereals for immune-boosting smoothies (almond milk and berries is a good combo), try organic spelt bread with nut butters or opt for organic eggs, tomatoes and mushrooms.

What you can do

- **Rinse it** 'When you are eating non-organic produce wash it in an acidic medium, made by adding one tablespoon of vinegar to a bowl of water. This will reduce some but not all pesticides,' says Patrick Holford.

- **Buy organic** Apples, celery, strawberries, blueberries, sweet bell peppers, peaches, nectarines, grapes, spinach, lettuce, cucumbers and potatoes form the 'dirty dozen' – fruits and vegetables with the highest toxic load. Avocados and mangoes are part of the 'clean fifteen'.

- **If it feels waxy, give it a miss** The resin used to coat fresh fruits and vegetables is sometimes made from shellac, derived from the secretion of lac bugs (yes, really!); you will sometimes even find this coating on organic foods according to Dr Campbell Douglass.[57]

- **Choose good-quality meat** Go for animal products that are organic and grass-fed, as well as antibiotic- and hormone-free. Better for the environment, the animal and you.

- **Avoid large, wild fish** Large predators such as swordfish, marlin, Chilean sea bass and tuna accumulate more mercury, so pick wild hake, herring, mackerel and sardines instead. And according to Dr William Campbell Douglass II, farmed fish should be permanently off the menu: 'Along with mercury, farmed fish can also contain PCBs and other chemical contaminants, as well as drugs such as antibiotics,' he says.

- **Keep up to date** Stay informed of the latest news by checking in with the Cancer Prevention and Education Society (www.cancerpreventionsociety.org) and Natural News (www.naturalnews.com).

At the Dentist

Some of the leading cancer centres in Europe won't accept patients until they have had their root canal teeth and mercury fillings removed. Mum stumbled across this fact when she was looking into various treatment centres following her diagnosis.

She had long known that mercury fillings were toxic – but root canals?

Dr Josef Issels, a German physician born around the turn of the twentieth century, believed that cancer was caused by weakening of the immune system and that root canals were often the culprit. The renowned doctor, who worked predominantly with terminal end-stage cancer patients, conducted a survey at his clinic and found that 98 per cent of adult cancer patients had serious oral-health problems. Issels would not initiate his successful treatments until all root canals had been removed.[58]

Recently, the Paracelsus Clinic in Switzerland published similar findings. In the years 1995–2000, Dr Thomas Rau who runs the clinic checked the records of the last 150 breast cancer patients admitted. He found that 147 of them (that's 98 per cent) had one or more root canal teeth on the same acupuncture meridian as the original breast cancer tumour. The Paracelsus Clinic[59] has three onsite biological dentists and all cancer patients have their mouth thoroughly cleaned and checked before starting treatment. This of course includes the removal of root canal teeth, if they correlate to the meridian of the cancerous organ. At Paracelsus they have the capacity to check the significance and toxicity of root canal treated teeth.

'We always remove root canals and fillings because they can trigger cancer,' reveals Dr Ursula Jacob. 'Root canals stimulate different acupuncture points in the body. So if a patient presents with liver cancer, we look at the correlating point in their mouth – just to check whether there is a root canal there.'

What is root canal therapy?

Root canal therapy (RCT) is sold as a treatment that can 'save' a decaying or dead tooth. But few patients are aware that the procedure comes with a lengthy list of possible side effects including cancer, sinusitis, multiple sclerosis, arthritis and eye disease.[60]

RCT involves clearing out and sterilising a dead tooth, filling it and then sealing it with a crown. The first problem with this is that it is impossible to sterilise a dead tooth, as reams of recent research now shows.[61]

'Part of the procedure of performing root canals is to disinfect the interior of the tooth over which there's still much controversy,' says Dr Diane Meyer, dentist, psychologist and author of *Pick Your Poisons*. 'Even in the natural health world there are dentists who say, "You can disinfect the root canal using laser" or, "You can disinfect it using ozone", but the fact remains that you still have this dead substance in the body.'

Based in Illinois, Dr Meyer is at the forefront of holistic dentistry. Following the realisation ten years ago, that her job – and her own amalgam fillings – were making her ill, she started researching and training with leading experts in natural health. Today, patients travel from around the globe – from as far afield as Australia and Japan – for Dr Meyer to repair their teeth and remove toxins that are sabotaging their health and well-being. On the subject of root canals Dr Meyer says: 'It sends off a lot of red flags to the immune system. When the nerve is removed from the tooth, it's dead. So the system now has to deal not only with this dead entity, but also bacteria that remain in the chambers.'

Over eighty-eight species of bacteria are found in dead teeth according to scientific literature, most of them anaerobic.[62] Dr Hal Huggins, a prominent dentist, author and researcher, illuminates just how dangerous this type of bacteria can be. In a lecture given to the Cancer Control Society in 1993[63] he explained that the bacteria within a dead tooth learn to live in the absence of oxygen, undergo a kind of mutation and produce thioethers – closely related to the chemicals used in mustard gas.

When I contacted Dr Huggins, who has received a Lifetime Achievement Award[64] for his work in biological dentistry, regarding the root canal/cancer link, the retired dentist had this to say: 'A lot has happened since 1993. We have done a fair amount of research on breast cancer and identified the top ten microbes from root canals that are found in the breast cancer patients.'

In addition to the toxins that leak from root canals (and studies show that *all* root fillings leak to varying degrees[65]), there is also the issue of what they are filled with. A veritable cornucopia of cancer-causing ingredients is poured into dead teeth – phenol, phenylmercury, formaldehyde, zinc oxide, to name a few. In Australia the most popular tooth cement for root canals is called AH26, which releases both formaldehyde and ammonia. It comes with the warning: 'Do not allow undiluted product or large quantities of it to reach ground water, water course or sewage system.' In other words, don't flush it down the loo, but by all means, insert it into your mouth.

Mercury fillings

If you can help it, don't live down-wind from a crematorium. In the UK up to 16 per cent of airborne mercury is estimated to be from crematoria burning fillings and teeth. Dental amalgam is not just an environmental hazard but a health hazard. As I mentioned earlier, there are 643 studies linking mercury with cancer and, according to Dr Garry Gordon, lead makes mercury up to 100 times more toxic.

In 2013 a new UN treaty was signed,[66] requiring countries to phase down the use of dental amalgam. This will put pressure on dentists worldwide to retrain in modern alternatives. Dr Meyer is part of a growing group of enlightened dentists who have found a better way: 'Silver amalgam fillings are classified as hazardous waste prior to placement in the body and hazardous waste after removal from the body,' she says, adding that eating or drinking hot items increases leaching from amalgam fillings, as does teeth grinding and chewing gum. When removing mercury fillings Dr

Meyer takes multiple precautions to ensure the individual, team and office are not poisoned. Some of these include supplying oxygen to the patient throughout the procedure and having no carpeting in the operating room to prevent mercury from embedding itself there. Along with adequate ventilation, negative ion generators are used to keep the air clean and mercury separators to ensure no waste-water contamination.

What you can do to protect your oral health

- **Change the tube** Stop brushing your teeth with toxins and opt for natural products instead. Both mum and I now use a 'tooth powder' containing simply myrrh, peppermint, baking soda, French grey sea salt, cinnamon, tea tree leaf, cranberry, vitamin C and a bioflavonoid complex.

- **Try oil pulling** This ancient Ayurvedic technique is used to cleanse and detoxify the whole body. 'The process is simply to swish unrefined oils (like coconut oil) throughout the mouth for several minutes,' explains Will Revak, holistic health educator and creator of the Healthy Mouth World Summit. 'Oil pulling gathers all sorts of debris like bacteria, fungi and viruses into the oil to be spat out.' One clinical study found that oil pulling substantially lowered the bacteria responsible for gingivitis[67] (early gum disease).

- **Get to know your teeth** Suffering from headaches or compromised digestion? Ever wondered whether your teeth might be involved? Will and Susan Revak have provided an interactive meridian tooth chart on their website where you can click on a specific tooth and see the internal organs associated with that tooth (www.orawellness.com/Videos/meridian-tooth-chart.html).

- **Investigate** If there's a dental substance you're not sure about, you can find out more through the Agency for Toxic Substances and Disease Registry.

- **Choose healthy bites** Certain foods can help strengthen tooth enamel and boost overall oral health. Ginger is known for its anti-inflammatory properties, seeds and nuts can help brush away plaque and pineapple can help remove stains from teeth thanks to the enzyme bromelain.

- **Find a holistic dentist**

At the Check-up

While prevention is certainly better than cure, we now know that mammograms and other routine scans are *causing* cancer, the very thing they are supposed to prevent.

A study released in 2009 found that computed tomography (CT) scans deliver up to four times more radiation than was previously believed.[68] Hot on the heels of that revelation came another study, led by the National Cancer Institute, showing that CT scans administered in the year 2007 alone may con-tribute to 29,000 new cancer cases and nearly 15,000 cancer deaths.[69]

Doctors rely heavily on CT scans to arrive at a 'definitive' diagnosis. But the images are not always what they seem, as anyone familiar with Suzanne Somers best-selling book *Knockout!* will know. This extract from the opening chapter reveals how the results from a CT scan led doctors to diagnose Somers with wide-spread cancer:

'The oncologist comes into my room. He has the bedside manner of a moose: no compassion, no tenderness, no cautious approach. He sits in the chair with his arms folded defensively.

"You've got cancer. I just looked at your CAT scan and it's everywhere," he says matter-of-factly. "Everywhere?" I ask, stunned. "Everywhere?"

"Everywhere," he states, like he's telling me he got tickets to the Lakers game. "Your lungs, your liver, tumours around your heart . . . I've never seen so much cancer."'

Following this traumatic news Somers was offered 'full-body chemo', which she refused. Instead she chose to have a biopsy which, in turn, revealed there was *no* cancer in her body: the CT scan had been misinterpreted.

The truth about mammograms

Next time a male physician insists you have a mammogram, you might want to borrow Arizona-based integrative oncologist Dr Thomas Lodi's cheeky reply: 'Let me ask you this: would you take your testicles, squash them and irradiate them?' Dr Lodi believes that a woman who starts getting 'recommended' mammograms every year in her thirties is almost guaranteed to develop breast cancer.

He's not the only one to take a strong position on this. 'Ten years of screening exposes you to about half the radiation you would have received had you been standing a mile away from the centre of the atomic bomb that destroyed Hiroshima,' says Lee Euler. 'If it weren't a medical test they'd call it murder.'

The conventional view

Chief Medical and Scientific Officer of the American Cancer Society, Dr Otis Brawley, recently said of mammography: 'Truth be told, it cannot avert all or even most breast cancer deaths.' Writing in the *Annals of Internal Medicine*, Dr Brawley also acknowledges numerous risk factors associated with mammograms including radiation exposure, breast compression pain, false-positive results, false-negative results, false-positive biopsy results and overdiagnosis.

What you can do

- **Have an ultrasound** 'Ultrasound reveals dense breast tumours better than mammography,' says Jenny Thompson, director of the US-based Health Science Institute. 'Ultrasound has one drawback. It can't confirm tumour malignancy. But in recent years, a technique called elastography changed all that. Elastography detects tumour flexibility. Benign tumours are soft and flexible. Malignant tumours are more rigid.'[70]

- **Opt for an MRI** 'They're excellent for finding invasive breast cancer and detecting the spread of cancer,' says Lee Euler. 'They can also "see around" breast implants and into the very dense breast tissue that's common in young women.' There's also evidence MRIs are more accurate than mammograms: in a study of 969 women at high risk for breast cancer, 121 tested positive for breast cancer with an MRI ... after receiving negative test results with mammogram.[71] Just to be clear, an MRI (magnetic resonance imaging) does not involve exposing the body to radiation. In fact, if the machine were to be tweaked slightly it could become very therapeutic, according to Dr Garry Gordon, who champions magnetic healing. And for the claustrophobic among us, there are now open, upright MRI centres available in the UK.

- **Find a thermographer** Thermograms are detecting breast cancer up to ten years earlier than mammograms. 'At least five important clinical studies in more than 300,000 women prove thermography is effectively detecting breast cancer in its early stages,' enthuses Lee Euler. This radiation-free procedure, which involves the clinician taking a thermal picture of the breast, has a growing number of supporters. Dr Bruce Rind, a leading holistic doctor based in Washington, explains why he believes it's the best choice: 'Mammograms only become useful once the cancer has been allowed to grow to a size the X-ray image can see,' says Rind. 'Thus a thermogram is like predicting the oncoming weather in one to two weeks, while a mammogram is to let you know how much it rained one to two weeks ago.' You will find more than 800 peer-reviewed studies on breast thermography in the medical literature.

On the Phone

We now check our mobiles every six and half minutes, according to a global study commissioned by Nokia,[72] and it's one of the many ways in which we increase our dose of dirty electricity. Wireless devices, cordless phones and computers all emit rays, referred to as either electromagnetic fields (EMF) or electro-magnetic radiation (EMR). These invisible rays disrupt cell communication and can wreak havoc on our health. 'Electro-smog both damages DNA and prevents your body from repairing DNA – which can be the first step to cancer,'[73] explains Marcus Freudenmann.

Wake-up call

A 2012 study published in the *Journal of Neuro-Oncology* showed that radiation from cell phones may damage DNA and alter genes in brain cells. The only thing more shocking than the research is the fact we've known about the dangers of mobile phones for thirty years: there are studies dating all the way back to the 1980s linking mobile phones to cancer.[74] Dr Andrew Davidson at the Fremantle Hospital in Australia studied the incidence of brain cancer in Australia from 1982 to 1992 and his research showed that cases of brain cancer doubled in that time,[75] while according to Patrick Holford, brain cancer is also on the increase in Britain and the US too. Dr Ursula Jacob has long warned of the dangers of cell-phone radiation and expects to see an increase in brain tumours, while Italian researchers found in 2011 that long-term mobile-phone use led to almost double the risk of head tumours.[76] Another study – from China – published in the journal *Cellular and Molecular Neurobiology* in 2012 shows that the microwave radiation emitted by mobile phones can transform normal cells into cancerous ones.[77]

Dizzying facts

In 2011 the World Health Organisation admitted that cell-phone radiation is a 'possible human carcinogen'.[78] Other 'possible human carcinogens' include chloroform, gasoline and the banned pesticide DDT.[79] One study cited in the WHO report showed a 40 per cent increased risk for gliomas (a type of tumour that starts in the brain or spine) among 'heavy users'. In other words, thirty minutes per day over a ten-year period.

Mobile-phone manufacturers are taking precautionary measures: when you buy a BlackBerry you'll now find, in small print, advice to keep phones at least 15mm away from the body to reduce your exposure to EMF.

What you can do

- **Turn it off** Whenever your phone or wireless internet is not being used, make sure it is switched off. And children and pregnant women 'should avoid talking on cell phones', writes Mark Hyman in the *Blood Sugar Solution.*

- **Avoid your hip** According to Hyman: 'The bone marrow in your hip produces 80 per cent of the body's red blood cells and is especially vulnerable to EMR damage.'

- **Don't use your mobile phone as an alarm clock** 'Buy an old style wind-up battery one for a few quid,' suggests Janey Lee Grace.

- **Check out green tea and bee propolis** 'A compound found within bee propolis, known as caffeic acid phenethyl ester (CAPE) has been experimentally tested to protect the kidneys, hearts and retinas of cell-phone exposed mice,' says Sayer Ji, founder and director of GreenMedInfo.com. 'EGCG, an antioxidant found in green tea, has also been shown to protect the liver against mobile-phone-induced radiation damage.'

- **Try medicinal mushrooms** 'In particular reishi and cordyceps protect tissues from radiation-related anoxia (oxygen deprivation), oxidative stress and inflammation, while detoxifying the body,' says integrative doctor and researcher Dr Isaac Eliaz.

- **Play detective** Wave a Trifield (an electrosmog detector) around your workspace or bedroom to check for areas high in EMFs. 'A reading of two is healthy,' explains Marcus Freudenmann, 'fifty to sixty shows serious electromagnetic disturbance.'

- **Buy a shield** There are now many products on the market which claim to protect you from radiation. Everyone in our family uses Green 8 EMF Radiation Protection Products which you can easily stick inside your mobile or underneath your home computer.

At the Hairdresser

It would be so much easier to turn a blind eye and enjoy the head massage, but the mounting evidence is making it hard to do so.

Over 5000 different chemicals are used in hair dye products alone, according to a quick comb through the research.[80] As we sip our lattes and read about Brad and Angelina, these toxins are rubbed into our scalps and inhaled, and some of them, like parabens, coal tar and lead acetate, are probable carcinogens.

Progressive dyes, which often contain lead acetate, must bear a large label cautioning people against using the product on their eyebrows and eyelashes, in their eyes, on their scalp if they have cuts or on any other parts of the body. Lee Euler sums up the message: 'Sounds like a lengthy way of saying, "Really, this stuff shouldn't come into contact with your body in any way whatsoever ... except the part you're willing to sacrifice for the sake of looking good".'

The National Cancer Institute (NCI) maintains the evidence is 'limited and conflicting' with regards to hair dye and cancer. None the less, it highlights a few key points:

- Studies show that people who started using hair dyes before 1980 have an increased risk of developing non-Hodgkin's lymphoma.

- Population studies have found an increased risk of bladder cancer in hairdressers and barbers.[81]

- Darker dyes are more harmful.[82]

Aside from hair dyes, there are obviously other factors worth teasing out. Weaves and hair extensions sometimes require acetone or formaldehyde-based removers,[83] 97 per cent of hair straighteners include petrochemicals,[84] and hair pomades and conditioners containing placental extracts have been linked to breast development in toddlers – according to Stacy Malkan, author of *Not Just a Pretty Face: The Ugly Side of the Beauty Industry.*

What you can do

- **Flush out toxins** 'If you're colouring your hair at home with a commercial dye, drink lots of water before during and after to protect the bloodstream and help flush out any unnecessary toxins,' says Terence Wilson, creative director and co-owner of Hair Organics in Notting Hill.

- **Dye it dirty** 'Don't shampoo your hair first as this will open up the pores in the scalp and cause irritation; and always do a skin test three to five days before,' cautions Wilson.

- **Hold that perm** Amy Cannon from Massachusetts recently won an award for developing a non-toxic perm using UV light to shrink-wrap hair. Watch this space.

- **Visit Skin Deep** This is the Environmental Working Group's cosmetic database which scores thousands of personal care products for toxicity.

In Your Handbag

Did you know there is likely to be lead in your lipstick,[85] mercury in your mascara[86] and arsenic in your antiperspirant deodorant? Or that some sanitary pads are lined with a dye that contains lead[87] and that tampons routinely contain traces of dioxins from bleach? These known carcinogens have been linked to hormone disruption and endometriosis.[88]

Mum has always considered herself fairly well versed in the

art of cosmetic chemical avoidance. As long as I can remember she has used shampoo free from sodium laureth sulfate, toothpaste free from fluoride and natural roll-on deodorants. Most products in our house, from the hand gel to the dog wash, are made by an American company that uses non-toxic ingredients. But like most women mum has her blind spots: the designer perfume she wore for twenty years, the occasional half a head of highlights, the anti-ageing face-creams ... All that changed last year, of course, when every potential carcinogen came under scrutiny, but for decades, mum practised a more relaxed policy when it came to her favourite beauty products.

I vividly remember standing at a beauty counter in Selfridges ten years ago as mum eagerly popped SK-II creams into her bag. These luxury skin-care products promised smooth, wrinkle-free skin, just like Cate Blanchett's. The secret ingredient, apparently, came via a Japanese monk who 'noticed that the workers in the sake brewery had extraordinary smooth hands'. Like millions the world over, mum was sold.

Fast forward to 2006, however, and a mob of smooth-skinned women were smashing doors at an SK-II branch in Shanghai, having just learned that their coveted products contain the toxic heavy metals chromium and neodymium. The manufacturer was quick to quell the furore. 'Procter and Gamble said the metals exist naturally, were not intentionally added to SK-II products and were safe at the low levels found in the products,' says Stacy Malkan. 'A few months later, the products were back on the shelves.'

The 'safe at low levels' argument has been trolleyed out by industry for as long as clued-up women have been asking questions. But it doesn't add up: 'The cosmetic companies typically don't consider the sometimes surprising impact of low-dose exposure, impacts on foetuses, chemical mixtures, interactions between genes and chemicals, or how deeply these products can penetrate,' says Malkan.

When we apply products to our skin they are absorbed immediately into our cells. Transdermal medications, like hormone creams, depend on this fact. A recent piece in the *New York Times* highlighted just how powerful skin products can be. The feature revealed that dogs and cats are now experiencing swollen breasts and hair loss thanks to their hormone-cream-wearing owners.[89]

In 2010 the US President's Cancer Panel report added fuel to the fire by suggesting that hormone-disrupting chemicals could be the source of many more cancer cases than previously thought. Scary when you consider that more than half of cosmetic products contain chemicals that can act like oestrogen or disrupt hormones.[90] The perfume bottle is where you're most likely to get your hit. At least 900 ingredients used to make fragrances have been identified as toxic, and a synthetic musk called galaxolide has recently been singled out for scrutiny: 'Trace amounts have been found in the fat, blood and breast milk of women who wear perfumes,' says Lee Euler. 'It's a known hormone disruptor, and some studies show that it may in fact contribute to the development of breast cancer.'

You might read all this with a knowing nod of the head, thinking, 'It's good to know, but I'm not going to change my beauty routine.' That's fine; we all have our sacred cows. But I would add that making changes isn't always about denial and compromise. When I discovered that my favourite beauty indulgence – fake tan (I'm ashamed to admit) – had a dark side, I was devastated. But on learning that diabetes, obesity, birth defects and cancer have been linked to the 'cocktail' of chemicals in bronzing lotions, I decided to look into alternatives. The upshot? I found Eco-Tan – an innovative new brand that contains no synthetic food colouring, GM ingredients or petrochemicals. And it's the most natural looking (and smelling) spray tan mum and I have ever had.

What you can do

- **Swap synthetic perfume for natural fragrance** The Organic Pharmacy recently released a range of 100 per cent natural and 85 per cent organic fragrances, containing cold-pressed essential oils. Mum stocks up on her favourite essential oil blends from Living Libations.

- **Keep nails natural** Next time you visit your high-street nail bar, BYO polish. 'Nail treatments are among the most toxic products on the Skin Deep base,' says Stacy Malkan. The brand, Butter London, has a covetable range of colours free of the 'evil three' (formaldehyde, toluene and DBP).

- **Ditch toxic tampons** 'There are feminine care options free of bleach, pesticides and toxic chemicals, including organic, unbleached tampons and pads,' says Malkan. Natracare is one non-toxic brand that's sold globally.

- **Make your own** Janey Lee Grace's book *Look Great Naturally . . . Without Ditching the Lipstick* is packed with easy-to-follow recipes.

- **Read labels** Check any suspicious ingredients on the Skin Deep website.

At the Airport

'Sit back, relax and enjoy the flight.' Announcements like this may soothe a fretful traveller, but no assurances can stop you being poisoned on a plane.

When you buckle your safety belt you are, in fact, strapping yourself in to a seat soaked in flame retardant. More specifically, a seat covered in the chemical called PBDE. In 2006 *National Geographic* magazine paid to have one of its workers – a journalist who flies thousands of miles each year as part of his job – tested for PBDEs. A chemical analysis revealed that the reporter's blood level of one particular PBDE was sky high, while levels of another were elevated enough to be considered high even for a factory worker making the chemicals.[91]

Gasping in horror? The in-flight air you breathe is also toxic. Once an aircraft flies above 3000 metres air has to be pumped into the fuselage since the air outside becomes thin with too little oxygen to keep people alive. In fact, 50 per cent of the air in an aircraft's cabin is bled off from the engine – and you wonder why you feel so lethargic after a long-haul flight? That vaporised jet oil contains neuro-toxic, immuno-toxic and potentially carcinogenic organophosphates.[92]

Flying also means being exposed to radiation: 'Cosmic radiation is a type of ionising radiation and originates from outer space and from our own sun,' explains Sheri Dixon, a UK-based mitochondrial therapist who became aware of cosmic radiation during her time working as a flight attendant. 'Studies have suggested that cosmic radiation may contribute to the development, over time, of certain cancers.' One study from the California Department of Health found that female flight attendants had a 30 per cent increased risk of breast cancer and twice the risk of malignant melanoma.[93]

What you can do

- **Go barefoot** 'As soon as you get off the plane, kick off your shoes and find some grass to ground yourself on,' says Marcus Freudenmann. Growing evidence suggests that connecting to the earth's surface plays a key role in keeping us healthy[94] (see Chapter 11).

- **Antioxidants for astronauts** 'A cosmonaut's body can age internally eight years for each year on earth, so it is imperative that they have access to all manner of radiation protection and shielding,' says Sheri Dixon, who sells carnosine-rich supplements developed for, and used by, Russian cosmonauts.

- **Vitamin C** 'I have Bio En'R-G'y C (see Chapter 4) and I drink it during the flight, and afterwards to help draw out the toxins,' says Freudenmann.

- **Say 'No' to body scanners** 'The scanners expose you to a significant amount of radiation,' says Lee Euler. The EU has already banned them and the American pilots' union has publicly advised members to opt for private pat-downs instead.[95] Don't be shy; be smart.

The Daily Detox

For serious detoxing, coffee enemas (Chapter 5), high-dose vitamin C (Chapter 4) and infrared saunas (Chapter 7) are unparalleled in their ability to clear out the system. However, there are also powerful supplements and super-foods that help pull poisons out of your body. Mum has experimented with all of them since her diagnosis, but as with everything in this book, what works for one person will not necessary work for the next. Here are just a few of them:

- **Seaweed** Not only are ocean plants packed with cancer-protective nutrients like magnesium and iodine, they are also natural detoxifiers: 'Alginates, found mainly in the Laminaria kelp species, have the

▶

---

ability to bind to toxins, heavy metals and dangerous radioactive particles in the digestive tract,' says Dr Isaac Eliaz, who specialises in natural removal of heavy metals.[96]

- **Wheatgrass** This 'flushes the blood, digestive system, and organs', writes Danica Collins in *The Top 10 Natural Cancer Cures*, while according to research by Dr Chiu Nan Lai of the University of Texas Health Sciences Center in Houston, wheatgrass is capable of reducing the carcinogenic effect of chemicals by up to 99 per cent.[97]

- **Coriander** This fragrant herb is a metal mobiliser and studies suggest it can stop lead accumulating in the body.[98]

- **Zeolites** These are negatively charged minerals derived from volcanic ash. According to Mike Adams, editor of *Natural News*, the zeolite crystal acts as a cage to trap toxic particles: 'It functions as a sort of dance club bouncer that captures free radicals, carcinogens and even viral particles, and tosses them out,' he writes. In one small preliminary trial zeolite was correlated with cancer remissions in 78 per cent of stage-4 cancer patients.[99] Dr Garry Gordon and Marcus Freudenmann are both big fans: 'I was completely mercury poisoned and zeolite changed my life,' says Freudenmann. 'When I started taking it in a sublingual form, my mind cleared up and my ability to concentrate improved dramatically. But as for my wife? She can't take it; it makes her feel unwell. So it's not for everyone.'

▶

- **Modified citrus pectin (MCP)** Derived from the pulp and rinds of citrus fruit, MCP removes poisons from the body and has been shown to halt the spread of cancer. In one study involving melanoma cells, MCP – administered intravenously – decreased tumour metastasis to the lungs by more than 90 per cent. The article was published in 1992 in the *Journal of the National Cancer Institute*.[100] Mum started taking MCP in powder form every morning for three months following her surgery.

From Paranoid to Proactive

We each have our own chemical load to contend with, based on our mother's womb, where we grew up and our current habits and lifestyle. Some of us are frequent flyers, others are regular Teflon fryers, some of us have an album of childhood X-rays, others have cupboards crammed with carcinogenic anti-ageing creams. There are things we can change, and things we cannot. But even if we succumb to convenience occasionally and order a non-organic plastic-wrapped takeaway, by having a solid detox routine in place, we can keep reasonably clean regardless (see 'The Daily Detox' box, above). 'I would have everyone you care about on a detoxification programme because the bottom line is, whether you're talking about autism, Alzheimer's, cancer or infertility, toxins are part of that problem,' says Dr Garry Gordon.

Our world has changed beyond measure and we need to upgrade our immune systems if we're going to thrive. However, it is important to remember that our inner world – our thoughts, our feelings, the memories we hold in our cellular tissue – will have as much influence on our health as any chemical concoction. So while it's worth taking the time to clean up your life, don't let paranoia ruin it. Make the necessary changes and then let go, remembering that a state of relaxation is the best environment in which to heal.

●

CHAPTER 7

Infrared Saunas and Hyperthermia

*'Give me a chance to create fever
and I will cure any disease.'*
Parmenides, Ancient Greek physician

If you ask a cancer patient to list the blessings that have come from their condition, they might be slow to touch on the good stuff. They might talk of the fear that now pervades their life – the endless check-ups and the side effects from treatment – before they get around to mentioning the love and support they've experienced, the things they no longer take for granted, the healthy habits they've adopted and the huge amount they've learned since their diagnosis. Cancer often triggers transformation – on a physical, emotional and spiritual level – and not only for the patient, but their family too.

As one of four children, it's been interesting for me to see how mum's experience has moved each of us to change in different ways. For my older brother Jeremy, the life and soul of the party, mum's diagnosis meant slowing down (a bit) and taking better care of his health: it meant getting a dog, getting married and stocking up on vitamins. For my little sister Emerald, it signalled time to move on. She realised that being healthy meant doing what you love, and a year after mum was diagnosed she quit her job as a corporate lawyer and moved to Paris to study cooking – *la vie est belle*. My little brother Banjo was still at university and living at home in Perth, when we discovered mum had cancer. He has been there to share some of mum's darkest moments and his quirky humour has kept her afloat. Being a bit of a carb-Nazi, Banjo has also helped mum cut down on her beloved pasta, while he, in turn, has cut down on dairy.

One thing we all have in common? We love hopping in mum's infrared sauna. When Christmas rolls around and we all head home, the hot seat is in high demand. 'Shotgun the sauna tomorrow morning,' my brother might say, while my sister and I agree to share it before going out – the sauna being the secret to party-perfect skin. Mum's sauna has become quite the social hub: her sister can often be found huffing her way through the recommended thirty minutes; other cancer patients stop by to de-robe and detox; and my brother sometimes watches an episode of *Game of Thrones* with his girlfriend, while in the sweat box.

It's long been known that heat can heal. From the Turkish hammam to the American Indian sweat lodge, traditional cultures around the world have used steamy spaces to purify the mind, body and spirit and modern research is now proving the benefit of sweating it out. Studies show that high temperatures help lower blood pressure,[1] eliminate toxins and boost white cell production and collagen growth.[2]

But while saunas are a fantastic way for cancer patients to keep their immune systems humming, when it comes to tackling cancer head on, hyperthermia is the hot ticket. This form of heat therapy has the ability to destroy tumours while leaving healthy cells intact.[3] And although mum hasn't tried the 'German miracle cure', as it's often referred to, thousands of others have. So in this chapter we take the temperature on a variety of heat therapies and explain how to get the most out of them.

Infrared Saunas

If you're tired of the treadmill, you might want to consider a few sessions in an infrared sauna. A recent American study found that you can burn up to 600 calories[4] in a thirty-minute stint. Saunas also help oxygenate the body: 'Saunas enhance circulation, which helps to bring essential nutrients, hormones and oxygen to the cells,' says Arizona-based integrative oncologist Dr Thomas Lodi. Cancer often shows up in poorly oxygenated areas of the body[5] (see Chapter 9), so improving circulation can be a vital part of the healing process.

Infrared heat is a form of energy that heats objects by a process called direct light conversion. It has nothing to do with the harmful UV rays associated with unprotected sunlight; in fact, infrared heat is so safe it's used in hospitals to warm newborn babies. The infrared spectrum consists of three wavelengths (near, mid and far). Many alternative cancer experts, including author and physician Dr Mark Sircus recommend using the latter: 'Far infrared heat reaches deeply into every area of the body. It increases cellular respiration so more toxins and wastes leave the cells,' he says. For the sake of simplicity, I will refer to far infrared (FIR) heat for the remainder of this chapter.

Get Moving

One of the easiest ways to sweat out toxins, improve lymphatic flow and reduce your risk of cancer – or recurrence – is exercise. 'If you really want to get well, as opposed to dreaming about getting well, exercise is not optional. It's mandatory,' says Lee Euler, author and publisher of the highly acclaimed newsletter *Cancer Defeated!* 'Multiple studies show it reduces the risk of cancer by half or more.'[6]

▶

As soon as mum recovered from her hysterectomy, exercise was put firmly back on the agenda. But she wasn't going back to her old routine. Rather than running herself ragged with a gruelling regime – Ashtanga yoga, followed by Pilates, power-plating and a vigorous daily dog walk – this time her focus was different. 'I now do exercise that doesn't overwhelm me, but makes me feel great,' mum says. Instead of worrying about weight loss, mum thought about what would make her body, mind and spirit feel lighter. She now took the time to check in, before working out. What did her body crave today? Did she feel like formal exercise or would her spirit be better served by a walk and swim at the beach?

With coffee enemas and vitamin injections to fit in, convenience became a priority for mum. That's when she discovered rebounding and shaking . . .

Jump around

Jumping on a mini tramp (rebounding) slows ageing, oxygenates the blood,[7] re-energises the brain and dramatically increases lymphatic flow. The lymph system helps remove toxins – such as dead cancerous cells, viruses and heavy metals – from the body, but unlike the blood (which is pumped by the heart) it takes physical movement to get fluids moving out of your lymph glands.

'Rebounding has been shown to increase lymph flow by up to thirty times,' writes Ty Bollinger in *Cancer – Step Outside the Box*. According to Lee Euler, one Mexican cancer clinic has a mini trampoline in every room, and they consider it one of the most important parts of their treatment protocol. Marcus Freudenmann, producer of the hit

▶

documentary *CANCER is Curable NOW*, is also a fan: 'Increasing lymph circulation by jumping gets white blood cells moving – critical for cleaning out your system and also killing cancer cells,' he says. 'Rebounding is especially good for those with breast cancer because it stimulates lymphatic drainage around the breast tissue.'

Shake it like a Polaroid picture

One of the more unusual additions to mum's new regime is shaking. For the last year, both mum and I have been shaking uncontrollably for twenty-four minutes, on a weekly basis. Renowned yoga teacher Gurmukh Kaur Khalsa (followers include Gwyneth Paltrow, David Duchovny and Madonna) believes shaking will fix 'every single thing': 'If you have disease, if you have depression, if you have anything going on that doesn't keep you in harmony with your divine self – gone, with the shaking,' declares Gurmukh in her DVD *Kundalini Yoga: Healthy Body Fearless Spirit.*

You don't need a gym membership or good weather to jump or shake for twenty minutes, and these are both simple, low-cost steps you can take to put your body back in healing mode.

Reducing your toxic load is crucial if you want to heal from cancer and saunas are a fantastic way to kick-start the process. A 2007 study from the American Environmental Protection Agency found that sauna therapy helps the body excrete lead, mercury, cadmium and fat-soluble chemicals such as PCBs.[8]

FIR saunas operate at a much cooler air temperature range

than their traditional counterparts: about 110–130°F (43.3–54.4°C) compared with 180–235°F respectively. Despite this, an FIR sauna is said to induce twice or three times the amount of sweat as conventional saunas, and you typically produce a sweat consisting of 20 per cent toxins in an FIR sauna, compared to only 3 per cent in a traditional one.[9]

Working up a sweat

Vietnam vets have been known to sweat out what looks like Agent Orange during an infrared sauna session:[10] 'It comes out in a brown sticky substance from under their arms,' says Mark Green, who works for Sunlight Therapies, an evidence-based complete wellness programme which includes a clinically tested brand of sauna. 'We've also had people who have, upon completion of their chemo and radium treatment, sweated out a black, unwashable, unmovable substance from their skin – you can't get it out of fabric.' Mark Green has witnessed first-hand the miraculous effects of sauna therapy. After contracting the debilitating Epstein-Barr virus (which can be a trigger for cancer[11]) and suffering from chronic fatigue for eleven years, Green heard about infrared saunas. A few weeks after an intense regime? Green felt well again. 'I went to my doctor and said, "Look I think this sauna is making me better, why would that be?" and he explained that blood-borne viruses cannot live outside the normal temperature range of human beings.'[12]

So how often should you hop in the sauna? Marcus Freudenmann advises cancer patients to aim for four or five sessions a week. 'You need to be in there for thirty to forty-five minutes and you should be soaking wet when you come out.' According to Freudenmann, if you're only getting a trickle down your cleavage you need to stick with it: 'Some people might need thirty sessions before they start really sweating. In other words, until you see sweat pouring from every part of your body – your head, your chest, your arms – the infrared sauna is not going to be doing its job.' To replace the lost fluids it's vital to drink plenty of (purified) water before and after a sauna. Hopping in a shower straight after a session is also recommended to remove toxins on the surface of the skin.

While you're in the hot box, Mark Green recommends drinking ginger tea. 'It raises your core temperature for higher and longer. It also cranks up your immune function and gives your liver a boost at the same time.' For Freudenmann, vitamin C is a sauna essential: 'When I have a sauna I take up to three heaped teaspoons of Bio En'R-G'y C in a litre glass bottle of water because you want to be sweating out as much as you can,' he says. 'I drink half the bottle before I go in and then the other part while I'm in the sauna, so the vitamin C can grab on to any toxins that don't make it out through the skin.'

Studies show FIR sauna treatment is safe, even for fragile patients. The renowned Mayo Clinic recommended it for thirty-four end-stage heart patients and their condition substantially improved.[13] However, it's advisable to check with your supervising practitioner before you embark on a regular sauna programme.

The best investment

FIR saunas don't come cheap. While you can find portable ones for less than £200, the stand-up two-seaters are likely to set you back at least £1000. Dr Sherry Rogers, author of *Detoxify or Die* puts the price into perspective: 'Insurance companies allow $100,000 for chemotherapy, radiation, bone-marrow transplants, tests and hospitalisations for the treatment of various types of cancer for which they know the median survival will be six months to five years at best. Paying $100,000 for no cure is not cost effective ... In contrast, with the far infrared sauna we are talking about reversing disease, getting rid of the underlying causes and therefore getting rid of the symptoms, once and for all.'[14]

While FIR saunas might be cost effective, you can't get past the fact they are prohibitively expensive for most. Thankfully, forward-thinking charities are stepping in to support proactive patients. The UK cancer charity Yes to Life offers grants to those hoping to add FIR saunas to their healing arsenal. 'Many cancer patients seek to use a sauna as a way of detoxifying through sweating, and as a low-level form of hyperthermia,' says Robin Daly, chairman of Yes to Life. 'Most users also report a greatly increased sense of well-being from regular use, which is a huge psychological boost among the rigours of cancer treatment.'

Forty-three-year-old Nicola, a breast-cancer survivor (who we met in Chapter 5), was able to buy an FIR sauna at a reduced price thanks to Yes to Life. 'I used it daily in the beginning and it really kick-started detoxification through my skin,' she says. 'I found that for the first time in my life I managed to sweat, especially when drinking plenty of water, and particularly when drinking at least two green juices a day. I used the sauna as part of a group of detoxification techniques: I might juice, then do an enema, then the sauna, followed by a hot/cold shower to get my lymph system going. I found that it really increased my thirst (which was a good thing, as I'd forgotten how to be thirsty and was very dehydrated). The whole family now uses it at the first sign of a cold.'

Mum purchased a two-seater sauna from Sunlighten[15] (after a dedicated campaign from her children). It looks like a deep-set wardrobe with a tiny slit in the glass door, perfect for those prone to claustrophobia. Mum uses time in the sauna to relax and unwind; the dimly lit space provides the perfect retreat from the outside world. But it also serves as a convivial cubby house to catch up with friends and family. 'Every Sunday was like a detox retreat in the house,' says my sister Emerald. 'Mum and I would have a gossip in the sauna, then she'd hop in a bath with bicarb soda [see Chapter 13] while I made us a juice.' These days when friends pop round mum flicks on the sauna rather than the kettle. Guests are only too eager to jump in the hot box and it saves mum the stress of not having any milk in the fridge (see Chapter 8).

If you are considering investing in an FIR sauna be sure to buy one which emits safe levels of EMF (electromagnetic fields). It turns out that most FIR saunas radiate dirty electricity to varying degrees, 'so it's essential that you check whether your brand offers low or NO EMF models',[16] says Freudenmann.

Hyperthermia

Hyperthermia is a kind of fever therapy where the temperature of the body is raised to the point where cancer cells self-destruct. Cancer patients who've been given weeks to live have travelled to Germany for this innovative treatment and returned cancer-free.

The fact that cancer cells 'can't take the heat' has been known for over a century. In 1868 Dr Peter Busch, a German–American doctor, found that one of his cancer patients miraculously recovered after suffering a raging fever. Since then, other cancer patients have experienced 'spontaneous remission' following a raised temperature,[17] including a British boy called Jordan Harden who had acute lymphoblastic leukaemia.[18] After both aggressive chemotherapy and an experimental stem-cell transplant failed, Jordan – only three years old at the time – was given weeks to live. In 2009 his parents were about to take him on a 'final' family holiday to Disneyland when they received news that Jordan no longer had cancer. Days before Jordan's final clear scans he'd had a temperature of 38.1°C (100.6°F). Could he have been cured by a fever?

The idea that high temperatures can selectively kill cancer

cells is no longer theory – it's fact. Numerous studies verifying the effectiveness of hyperthermia can now be found on the National Cancer Institute[19] website, and clinical trials are currently under way at leading research institutes including the University of California.[20] But the Germans are way ahead of the game: 'Twenty years ago, we had the biggest hyperthermia centre in Europe,' says integrative oncologist Dr Ursula Jacob. 'We had about 100 beds in the clinic and over the years we saw that hyperthermia not only mobilised the immune system, but also improved long-term survival.'

In 2009 Munich-based Professor Rolf Issels presented impressive results from a 341-patient study of hyperthermia. Issels found that adding hyperthermia[21] to chemotherapy reduced the risk of cancer recurrence or death by 42 per cent. In addition, tumour shrinkage occurred in just 12.7 per cent of patients assigned to chemotherapy alone as opposed to 28.8 per cent assigned to the combination therapy.[22]

How it works

'Hyperthermia helps the immune system to recognise and destroy tumour cells,' says Dr Jacob. Dr Alexander Herzog, head of Dr Herzog's Special Hospital[23] near Frankfurt explains the process in more detail: 'The treatment helps to develop heat shock proteins on the surface of the tumour cells, making them more visible to the attacks of the immune system.' In this chapter we look at three of the most promising forms of hyperthermia and give you a glimpse of what it's like to be in the hot bed.

Local hyperthermia

More gentle than whole-body hyperthermia, local hyperthermia involves heating up one area of the body – such as the breast, cervix or stomach. It is also used when the cancer is not widespread: 'So we would use local hyperthermia if the cancer has spread to the liver, for example, but not other organs,' explains Dr Herzog. At Herzog's Special Hospital the heat is applied using radio-wave frequencies. Temperatures higher than 42°C (107.6°F) are achieved in the cancerous tissue, but only malignant cells are damaged. 'With local hyperthermia, the patient is awake and they don't feel anything because the skin is cooled down by an applicator,' explains Herzog. 'So the tissue heats up, but you don't feel it ... most patients fall asleep during the procedure.'

For Nicola, the treatment was pain-free, but not necessary relaxing. 'I had local hyperthermia in the axilla area [near the underarm],' she says. 'I couldn't feel the heat, which was very targeted, but it was quite uncomfortable to get into a position and hold it for twenty minutes. I had it in conjunction with high-dose vitamin C infusions (sometimes with hydrogen peroxide), so I always felt amazing afterwards – lots of energy, a bit invincible. Looking back, although it was difficult at the time, I would definitely do it again.'

Nicola's physician was Dr Siegfried Trefzer from the Hightree Medical Clinic in Sussex, England. 'Local hyperthermia is not just for cancer patients,' stresses Trefzer. 'It can also be very helpful for things like rheumatoid arthritis, frozen shoulder, auto-immune disease, Raynaud's, fibromyalgia – and most conditions that are caused by poor circulation,' he says. However, hyperthermia is best known for treating, and sometimes reversing, cancer.

In Holland, local hyperthermia, combined with radiation, is currently the standard treatment for advanced cervical cancer.[24] Commenting on the success of this combination, Herzog says: 'With advanced cervical cancer you typically have a cure rate of less than 20 per cent, but when you add in hyperthermia, those rates improve up to 50 or 60 per cent – that's a big difference.'

Whole-body hyperthermia

In this instance the patient's entire body is heated for four to five hours. Marcus Freudenmann has witnessed dozens of German doctors administer this treatment, often with 'stunning' results. 'Full-body hyperthermia is often used in the late stages, when the patient has metastases all over their body,' says Freudenmann. The doctors ramp the heat up to 41.5, 41.8 which is pushing what your body can stand. But if you bring a person to that stage you can kill cancer cells.' Lee Euler has interviewed dozens of doctors and cancer survivors in Germany: 'There's Vida, a forty-five-year-old woman with a giant tumour in her lung. She underwent this treatment – and within six weeks her tumour had disappeared. The fever therapy also saved forty-two-year-old Dieter from stomach cancer fourteen years ago. He's fine today,' he says.

During whole-body hyperthermia patients are put to sleep using sedation. Following the session, they might feel tired – 'like you might feel after a high fever,' explains Herzog; 'but then you would be feeling normal by the next day.' In about 30 per cent of cases, whole-body hyperthermia might result in blisters on the lip and 'puffiness'. 'The fever blisters take about one or two weeks to resolve, like normal cold sores,' says Herzog. 'The puffiness usually disappears within twenty-four hours and then a very small number of patients – maybe 2–4 per cent of cases – might have superficial blisters or burns at the skin level, which might take longer to heal.'

Hyperthermia for prostate cancer

'If I had any stage of prostate cancer – early or late – personally, I'd forget about the "home remedies" and go straight to Germany, because their top method of treatment is extremely effective when it comes to curing prostate tumours,' says Lee Euler.

One of my blog subscribers, Lance from Adelaide, Australia, did just that. When he was diagnosed with prostate cancer, aged seventy-one, he eschewed conventional treatment and travelled to Klinik St Georg. 'A lot of my friends have had prostate surgery and I know about all the horrible side effects – you hear about them becoming incontinent and walking around wearing nappies,' he says. 'So I sent away for various books, and I heard about all these different clinics in Europe and in Mexico – eventually, I came across Klinik St Georg. I stayed for a fortnight and had two sessions of prostate hyperthermia, lasting three hours each.'

So what does the therapy involve? A catheter is inserted into the prostate with an electrode attached. This electrode then emits a radio wave which heats up the prostate. Sound like medieval torture? Fear not: 'The doctors turn the switch on and it's totally painless,' says Lance. 'You just sit there while the machine does its electronic wiz-bo; you can't feel anything. It also kills any fungus and mould that's been there for years. So you come out as clean as a whistle and like an eighteen-year-old again!' The result? 'My PSA [Prostate Specific Antigen] was 48 before I left Australia, and when I came back it was 0.1. My PCA 3 test [a marker for prostate cancer] confirmed the cancer was gone. Twelve months before having hyperthermia the reading was 37 and when I came back from Germany it was 4.'

Lance's is just one of many success stories to come out of Klinik St Georg. 'Since 1992, we have treated thousands of prostate patients, especially prostate cancer, and we did not have to do surgery in a single one,' says the eminent integrative oncologist Dr Friedrich Douwes. 'Most of the patients are cancer-free for the next ten years.'

Keep your hair on

The devastating side effects from chemotherapy are often greatly diminished when used alongside hyperthermia: 'You don't lose your hair and the chemotherapy works much more effectively,' says Marcus Freudenmann. Many practitioners, including Dr Ursula Jacob, choose to use a lower dose of chemotherapy thanks to these synergistic effects. At the Special Hospital, Dr Herzog uses two types of whole-body hyperthermia – one with chemotherapy and one without: 'With the extreme whole-body hyperthermia, you reach temperatures of 41°C or higher; in this case you use the thermic effect of hyperthermia to enhance the efficacy of the chemotherapy,' he says.

If the patient doesn't want chemotherapy, Dr Herzog would use something called 'moderate' hyperthermia, which involves heating the body to 39 or 39.5°C (102.2 or 103.1°F) and requires only light sedation. 'Here we use the fever effect to stimulate the immune system in a very intensive way,' he says. The immune-boosting effects of hyperthermia are well known: 'It stimulates the production of interleukin 2 which, in turn, mobilises natural killer cells,' says Dr Ursula Jacob.

Hyperthermia also improves the efficacy of natural treatments including artemisinin (Chinese Woodworm), oxygen and high-dose vitamin C. Lee Euler explains why the latter is such a dynamic duo: 'Any cancer cells that remain after the hyperthermia are so weak that another therapy such as vitamin C can kill them off.'

What kind of cancers will hyperthermia work for?

Herzog reports excellent results with breast, cervical, colon and ovarian cancers. 'Certain lymphomas respond well, as do stomach cancers and sarcomas,' he adds. In patients with advanced metastatic breast cancer (spread to the bones) Herzog and his team have published success rates of 70–80 per cent when hyperthermia is used alongside chemotherapy: 'These success rates are very high – much higher than all other combinations published,' says Herzog. However, he is quick to temper any hype over the results: 'Success doesn't mean cure, by the way,' he says. 'It means that the patient goes into remission, which can be a complete remission – meaning the cancer is completely gone – or partial remission, which means the cancer is gone partly; or it could even mean "disease control", so the cancer is not growing any more.' It's difficult for doctors to predict the outcome for patients: 'We see patients who have had many treatments before they come to us, which lessens the likelihood of success,' admits Herzog, 'but even in those cases, we have astonishingly high numbers of success.'

When he was diagnosed with liver cancer Voyt Reich, one of my blog subscribers from Brisbane, Australia, didn't think he had much hope. But one year after visiting Dr Herzog his tumours are shrinking. 'When my hepatologist told me I had a few weeks to live I was devastated, but somehow my inner voice was telling me that he was wrong,' says Voyt, who was so inspired by his trip to Germany he decided to set up his own integrative cancer clinic in Kuala Lumpur along with two Malaysian physicians. 'That way Australians will only have to fly eight hours instead of twenty-four!' he says.

Hyperthermia has gained a reputation as the therapy to try when all else fails, and Dr Garry Gordon, co-founder of the American College for Advancement in Medicine (ACAM), swears by it: 'If a patient has cancer that is so out of control they're supposed to die in ten days – if it's in every part of their body, they're living on IV morphine – if they have the money, I would fly them directly to Munich and I would suggest they go to see Dr Douwes to have hyperthermia.' Dr Friedrich Douwes has worked with cancer patients since the 1970s and has been using natural treatments alongside conventional medicine for the last thirty years.

Need to know

Detoxification is important before embarking on hyperthermia, according to the experts: 'Free radicals will sidetrack the immune system from the real challenge,' says Dr Trefzer, who believes treatments are more effective if the patient has done some sweating, exercise and fasting beforehand. At Klinik St Georg patients are also primed before they begin hyperthermia: they are routinely given intravenous vitamins and minerals such as zinc and selenium to improve their condition. 'If your toxic load is high and your methylation process isn't functioning properly, hyperthermia won't increase your healing probabilities very much,' emphasises Marcus Freudenmann.

While hyperthermia is far from being widely available, the wheels are in motion across the continents – from Canada to Japan – and it's proving particularly popular among Australians. In 2012 an 'oncothermia' clinic was opened at the Prince of Wales Hospital in Sydney, and in Melbourne the National Institute of Integrative Medicine (NIIM) is currently studying the effects of hyperthermia when used in conjunction with chemotherapy and radiation.[25] As testament to the growing demand for cutting-edge alternative therapies, even the *Australian Financial Review* decided to cover hyperthermia in their December 2012 issue. The article came with the following introduction: 'Nothing annoys some readers of this page more than yet another story on the conventional management of prostate cancer. They have lost faith in this process and believe too many men are suffering the consequences of being overtreated. Some question the basic assumptions and say the treatment paradigm is flawed. After receiving innumerable emails and letters from readers on this subject, Jill Margo devotes her last column of the year to three such readers who don't believe the disease is being appropriately managed in Australia.'

In our myopic quest for 'a cure', are we missing opportunities to heal? Rather than aiming to annihilate every cancer cell, would it not be better to focus on feeling better? 'Our principal aim is to make sure that the treatment of cancer should not harm the patient more than the disease does already,' says Dr Herzog.

'The quality of life is one of our most important aims. Every day lived with joy is of infinite value.' Herzog believes that cancer is a chronic disease which requires constant monitoring: 'Hyperthermia is not a cure, so maybe at some time the cancer becomes active again and we have to start a second attempt. But we have patients for many years who return for follow-up treatments and the treatments work and work again,' he says.

Of course, hyperthermia will not work for everyone. Mum has lost two friends to cancer while I have been writing this book. Both travelled to Germany as a last resort, and sadly, it didn't work out for them. As Caroline Myss puts it in *Why People Don't Heal And How They Can*: 'Sometimes it's just time for the spirit to be called home.'

Despite inspiring testimonies and impressive success rates, no doctor can tell you how your own journey will unfold. But that's not to say you should abdicate responsibility and leave your health in the hands of fate. Rather, weigh up all your options, consider the cost/benefit analysis of every treatment (both financially and physically) and know that for every dire prognosis, there is someone who has defied it: so why not you?

●

CHAPTER 8

There's Something About Dairy

'In my view, anyone with cancer should
give up dairy completely.'
Dr Patrick Kingsley, author of *The New Medicine*

I f there's one thing guaranteed to spark heated debate, it's discussing the perfect diet for cancer patients. Many practitioners
believe it's vital to give up animal protein; others say organic
meat helps patients thrive. Some experts say patients must avoid
carbs at all costs; others are big on brown rice. For some doctors,
cold food compromises digestion and weakens immunity; for
others raw food is the only way.

But there is one message that seems almost universal: give up
dairy. Here is just a smattering of advice from world leading
cancer experts:

'Most hormonal cancers are related to milk, I believe'
Dr Tsuneo Kobayashi, Japanese oncologist

'You have to give up the wheat and dairy –
these are obvious things'
Dr Garry Gordon, Co-Founder of the American College
for Advancement in Medicine (ACAM)

*' Get rid of dairy . . . and get rid of margarine for
Christ's sake'*
Dr Zenon Gruba, Australia-based practitioner

So after the third practitioner insisted dairy was bad news, mum made the decision to give it up entirely. But it wasn't easy. In our household, a cup of hot tea with milk has long been the answer to life's setbacks, big and small. When the air is thick with anxiety and fear, the best way to fill the silence is to fill the kettle; it was the first thing mum did when she returned from the hospital following her hysterectomy.

But when she finally gave dairy the flick? Her stomach flattened, her skin glowed and she wondered why she hadn't done it years before.

The Dairy–Cancer Link

In 2003 British scientist Professor Jane Plant caused a media sensation with the release of her book *Your Life in Your Hands*. Her message – that breast cancer can be treated and prevented with the right food – was met with worldwide acclaim. The book documents how Plant herself beat cancer (five times) and how making one simple dietary change was the key to her recovery.

Plant was diagnosed with breast cancer in 1987. She underwent conventional treatment including a radical mastectomy, thirty-five radiotherapy treatments and twelve sessions of chemotherapy – and was told she had three months to live. 'I was so upset, I asked the doctors to just give me an injection and put me down,' says Plant. 'Positive thinking wasn't there at all . . . but then I heard my son asking for me and that sort of made me get my act together.' Plant was forty-two years old when she first noticed the lump on her breast; six years later the disease had spread to her lymph system.

'I was left with a large lump the size of half a boiled egg sticking out of my neck,' says Plant. 'The latest round of chemotherapy was having no effect on this lump; I was measuring it with calipers, so I knew.'

But the life-saving epiphany came when her husband, Peter, also a scientist, returned from a trip to China. 'We were musing on why so few Chinese women got breast cancer and suddenly it struck me that they didn't have any dairy products in their diet,' says Plant.

According to 2008 figures[1] the incidence of breast cancer for women in China is 21.6 for every 100,000; in America the rate is 76, in Australia it's 84.8, in the UK it's 89.1 and in France – a country famous for its love affair with butter and cream – it's 99.7.

Plant knew these differences weren't genetic, since migrational studies demonstrate that when Chinese or Japanese people move to the West the rates of breast (and prostate) cancer go up. 'In China they call breast cancer "Rich Women's Disease" and when you asked the people what that meant they said it was, "people who eat Hong Kong food" – in other words, Western food,' says Plant.

Within days of her giving up dairy the malignant lump on Professor Plant's neck had begun to shrink and within six weeks it had vanished completely. Her cancer, deemed incurable, has not returned since. Since Plant's remarkable recovery twenty-five years ago, there has been an avalanche of research pointing to the dangers of consuming dairy.

Live Eight Years Longer?

Dr Joe Esposito, lecturer, health consultant and author of *Eating Right ... For the Health Of It!* says: 'A study done not so long ago showed that if you stop eating dairy products you have an average of eight quality years added to your life.' According to Dr

John A. McDougall, an American physician and nutrition expert, the dangers of dairy are manifold: 'Heart disease, cancer, type-2 diabetes, arthritis and infectious disease are only a few of the common consequences of drinking milk from other animal species,' he says. Others agree. In his book *Devil in the Milk* Dr Keith Woodford refers to over 100 published, peer-reviewed papers revealing that substances in milk have been linked to type-1 diabetes, heart disease, autoimmune disorders, autism and schizophrenia.[2]

But nowhere is the research more persuasive than on the subject of cancer: 'There is now consistent and substantial evidence that the higher the milk consumption of a country, the greater their breast and prostate cancer risk,' says British nutritionist and author Patrick Holford. 'The highest risk of cancer death is found in Switzerland, Norway, Iceland and Sweden, countries that are among the biggest consumers of milk.'

Dairy might be particularly bad news for ovarian cancer. In one Swedish study consumption of lactose and dairy products was positively linked to ovarian cancer.[3] In addition, a study conducted in Denmark (where the incidence of ovarian cancer is one of the highest in the world) found that for women who consumed more than two servings of milk per day the risk of developing ovarian cancer was nearly twice that of women who drank less than half a serving per day.[4]

Boosting Gut-friendly Bacteria

While products like Activia have raised awareness about the importance of probiotics, many people remain unaware there are non-dairy alternatives – or that these alternatives have been around for thousands of years.

Kimchi, made from fermented vegetables, is Korea's

national dish, natto and tempeh (forms of fermented soya bean) have long been staples of the Japanese diet and sauerkraut can still be found on hot dog stands throughout Eastern Europe. Made from pickled cabbage, sauerkraut is one of the best food sources of vitamin C and great for balancing intestinal flora.

New takes on old 'cultures' are cropping up everywhere thanks to the burgeoning vegan market. Donna Gates, nutritionist, lecturer and author of *The Body Ecology Diet*, recently created her own non-dairy fermented drink, which she describes as 'champagne like'. The drink, CocoBiotic, is made from wildcrafted young Thai coconut and organic kefir grains. 'Everybody needs to have fermented foods in their diets,' says Gates. 'The microflora in our gut manufacture B vitamins – B3, B6 and B12 – as well as vitamin K. They also help regulate hormones like oestrogen, protect us from parasites and stimulate our immune system.'

Research shows that up to 80 per cent of the body's immune system is located in and around the gut. These 'good bacteria' that reside deep in our belly play a vital role in recognising and communicating what we need to stay healthy. 'The gut wall is another brain inside the body and is connected to the brain in our head,' says Gates. Friendly bacteria play a key role in regulating our immune system and probiotics are known to help fight cancer. 'They increase antibody response[5] and enhance natural killer function,'[6] says Gates. In studies looking at colon cancer cells, probiotics were shown to inactivate carcinogens that can damage DNA[7] and produce compounds that prevent cells from mutating. In a separate study, healthy bacteria were shown to produce enzymes that help break down pesticides[8] and other toxic chemicals like BPA.[9]

Then there's prostate cancer. According to the National Cancer Institute (NCI), nineteen out of twenty-three studies have shown a positive association between dairy intake and prostate cancer,[10] and if you have a family history of colorectal cancer you might want to pore over research uncovered by Patrick Holford. In 1937, a group of 4999 children in the UK took part in a long-term study recording their dietary habits year on year. 'Some sixty-five years later,' says Holford, 'those with a high dairy intake during childhood were found to have tripled their odds of having colorectal cancer.'[11]

Why Milk Feeds Cancer

'Milk contains thirty-eight different hormones and growth pro-moters,' explains Patrick Holford. 'But one in particular is attracting a lot of attention. It's called insulin-like growth factor, or IGF-1.' IGF-1 naturally circulates in our blood and, like cortisol, proges-terone and oestrogen, it's an important and necessary hormone – it's in mother's milk to ensure the baby grows, and levels of IGF-1 rise in puberty to stimulate the growth of breasts. But as we grow older, levels naturally drop off. That is, unless you're a dairy lover.

'We certainly know that people who consume a lot of dairy products will have higher levels of IGF-1,'[12] says Holford. 'It also stimulates the body to produce more of its own. It simply does what it's meant to do – stimulate growth. It also stops over-growing cells from committing suicide, a process called apoptosis.' Given that the main aim of chemotherapy drugs is to *stimulate* apoptosis, any substance that hinders this process is bad news. 'IGF-1 is one of the most powerful promoters of cancer growth ever discovered for cancers of the breast, prostate, lung, and colon,'[13] says Dr John McDougall. 'Overstimulation of growth by IGF-1 leads to premature ageing too – and reducing IGF-1 levels is "anti-ageing",'[14] he adds.

But What About My Bones?

We've been repeatedly told that drinking milk builds strong bones, but clinical research tells a different story. One study which followed more than 72,000 women for eighteen years showed no protective effect of increased pasteurised milk consumption on fracture risk.[15] Another study, published in the *Archives of Pediatrics & Adolescent Medicine*, found that adolescent girls consuming the most dairy products and calcium had *no* added bone protection. The seven-year study found that among the most physically active girls, those who got the most calcium in their diets (mostly from dairy products) had more than double the risk of stress fractures.[16]

Patrick Holford is adamant that *nobody* needs dairy in their diet: 'If you look at population studies there is no correlation between calcium intake, dairy intake and osteoporosis,' he says. 'Half of the world's populations don't consume dairy products and they are fine. So if an individual chooses to not have dairy products, but is eating beans, nuts, seeds, vegetables and so on, there is no reason why they shouldn't continue to get enough calcium.' There's another benefit to choosing non-dairy foods: 'Eating nuts, seeds and greens gives you the right balance of calcium and magnesium but you *don't* get that balance in dairy products,' says Holford.

So where has this message that we need milk for calcium come from? 'Calcium deficiency is a commercial ploy to sell you more calcium pills and dairy products,' says McDougall. In America, the National Dairy Board has spent over $1.1 billion to promote dairy products, and milk is the second-largest agricultural commodity in the US.[17] In other words, dairy is big business and financial factors largely drive the 'drink milk' message. The very definition of milk could even be subject to change if the International Dairy Foods Association and the National Milk Producers Federation have their way. They have filed a petition with the US FDA to alter the definition of 'milk' to include chemical sweeteners such as aspartame and sucralose. In other words, none of these additives would need to be listed on the label.[18]

The Raw Truth

Economic factors also figured in the landmark decision to pasteurise milk over a hundred years ago. Pasteurisation not only dramatically increases the shelf life of milk, but it also takes the power and profit away from the dairy farmers themselves. Rather than selling their milk at market price direct to consumers, farmers are essentially forced to sell their product to milk processors, which buy the milk from them to sell on to supermarkets at a fraction of its value.

Unpasteurised (or 'raw') milk vanished from our diets in the 1950s when pasteurisation became the norm – along with lactose intolerance. The aim of pasteurisation, which involves heating milk to 72 degrees, is to kill any pathogens; but this process also destroys vital nutrients, including the beneficial bacteria, lactase, necessary to digest lactose. 'In my practice, many patients can't tolerate pasteurised milk, but they are able to tolerate raw milk,' says integrative health practitioner Chris Kresser.[19]

Raw milk also contains disease-fighting antibodies and fat-soluble vitamins A, D and E that pasteurisation alters by up to 66 per cent. Primitive cultures around the world have long been aware of the immune-boosting benefits of drinking raw milk. The traditional diet of the African Maasai consisted of nothing more than meat, blood and raw milk. Nutrition pioneer Dr Weston Price described the Maasai people as being characterised by 'superb physical development, great bravery and . . . superior intelligence'.

We've been told that it's necessary to pasteurise milk to destroy all of the bacteria, but if you think pasteurisation guarantees protection against pathogens – think again. In the last few decades there's been a stream of outbreaks linked to heat-treated dairy. In America, between 1982 and 1997, 220,000 people contracted salmonella from pasteurised milk[20] and in 2007 three people in New England died from drinking bacteria-contaminated pasteurised milk.[21] Of course, as with any food, some people *do* get sick from drinking raw milk, but the risk is minute according to experts: 'The absolute risk of developing a serious illness – one that would require hospitalisation – from drinking raw milk is exceedingly small,' says Chris Kresser. 'It's about one in six million.'

Pus Cells in Your Milk?

If you don't believe processed dairy is dirty, consider this FDA ruling: you cannot have more than 750,000 pus cells per ml of milk or you can't sell it. This means that a 240ml glass of conventional pasteurised milk may contain up to 180 million pus cells. 'In 2011, the dairy industry debated lowering the allowable level of pus cells (somatic cells) to just 450,000 per ml,' according to Health Ranger Mike Adams, 'but it chose to keep the levels at 750,000, allowing for more infections and more pus in the pasteurised milk sold at grocery stores everywhere.'[22]

As for raw dairy farmers, they *must* comply with strict regulations: 'We're inspected regularly – and tested regularly – so it has to be clean,' says Dave Paul, a third-generation farmer who sells raw milk at local markets in London. Paul's cows are fed on grass, provided with clean housing and the milk is cooled down to three degrees within a quarter of an hour of the cow being milked.

Raw Dairy: Cancer Protective or Cancer Provoking?

In its natural state, milk may have some anti-cancer benefits: 'The whey proteins in raw milk boost glutathione,' says Chris Kresser. 'But when you pasteurise milk it denatures the whey proteins so they're not able to raise glutathione levels.' Kresser refers to glutathione as a 'bullet-proof vest' – not only does this anti-oxidant neutralise free radicals, it also boosts natural killer cells and detoxifies the liver (see Chapter 5).

But although raw milk provides a host of immune-boosting benefits, there is no getting around the fact that it contains IGF-1. 'I would fully expect IGF-1 levels to be high in goat's milk, organic milk and raw milk,' says Patrick Holford. 'The point with IGF-1 is that it's known as a cancer cell growth promoter, but not an *originator*; in other words, I don't know of any evidence that dairy *causes* a normal cell to become a cancer cell, I just know that it does encourage cancer cells to grow faster,' he says.

If you've been diagnosed with cancer, you might not want to take your chances with this one. 'I recommend the complete avoidance of dairy products,' says Holford. 'If you don't have cancer, keep your intake of dairy products low.' Holford encourages non-cancer patients to experiment going dairy-free for a week and seeing how they feel: 'You may find relief from some niggling symptoms you have suffered from in the past. If you find your indigestion or bloating stops, the headaches you have suffered from have stopped, your energy increases or your sniffs and snuffles clear up, get yourself tested for dairy intolerance,' he says.

Switch to Soya?

This is one of the most divisive issues in the world of holistic health. On the one hand, we know that Asian cultures –

traditionally big consumers of soya – have lower rates of breast, prostate and colon cancers; but on the other hand, modern soya products have been shown to depress thyroid function,[23] cause reproductive problems (in men and women), increase heart disease, lower libido and *increase* the risk of certain cancers.

In July 2005 researchers at Cornell University's Program of Breast Cancer and Environmental Risk Factors warned that excessive soya food consumption can increase breast cell multiplication, putting women at greater risk for breast cancer. In the same year the Israeli Health Ministry warned that babies should not receive soya formula, that children under eighteen years of age should not eat soya foods more than three times a week and that adults should exercise caution because of the adverse effects on fertility and increased breast cancer risk.[24]

One of the most outspoken critics of soya is Dr Kaayla T. Daniel, author of *The Whole Soy Story: The Dark Side of America's Favorite Health Food*. 'Respected scientists have warned that possible benefits should be weighed against proven risks,' she says, adding that the phytoestrogens (oestrogen-like chemicals found in plant foods) in soya are strong enough in numbers to cause 'significant endocrine disruption'. However, many practitioners, including Patrick Holford, strongly believe the phytoestrogens serve to balance hormone levels. Professor Plant is also a soya supporter. She explains that the plant oestrogens in soya protect the breast in the same way as Tamoxifen (a drug that blocks the action of oestrogen).

Good soya, bad soya

While the relative benefits of soya will no doubt continue to be debated for some time, what we know for sure is that Asian cultures haven't been sipping highly processed, genetically modified soya milk for centuries.

'Asians eat different soya foods from the ones now appearing on the Western table,' says Dr Kaayla Daniel. 'Think small amounts of traditional whole soya foods such as miso, natto, tempeh, tofu, tamari and shoyu – not veggie burgers, 'energy bars', shakes, TVP chili, soya milk or other meat or dairy substitutes.'

Fermented soya products have been shown to lower cholesterol and blood pressure and inhibit cellular mutations. Indeed, one fermented soya beverage, Haelan 951 (see box), has been shown to reverse some stage-4 cancers where other treatments could not.

Haelan 951: the Fermented Soya Beverage That Kills Cancer Stem Cells

Eighteen months after her diagnosis mum travelled to Germany to get the scoop on the best alternative treatment for her, based on a molecular blood analysis (see Chapter 10). It turned out to be a product she'd never heard of: Haelan 951.

Over the last twenty years the fermented soya beverage has shown that it will significantly improve a cancer patient's clinical condition and quality of life. Dr Morton Walker, author of ninety-two books including fourteen bestsellers and winner of twenty-three medical journalism awards, believes it may be the 'best nutritional supplement'. He has interviewed around a hundred patients who claim Haelan is the only cancer treatment that has helped their return to health.

Haelan targets cancer at its source, by taking on cancer stem cells. It's estimated these cells account for less than 1 per cent of any original cancer tumour[25] – but don't be

▶

fooled. These highly aggressive, slow-growing cells are the ones that kill the patient. 'Chemotherapy and radiation do not kill cancer stem cells[26] – they only selectively kill the non-malignant cells in the tumour,' says Walter H. Wainright, the world's foremost authority on Haelan. 'In addition, all cancer cells start to mutate within two hours of being hit with chemotherapy,' he adds.

Research suggests the fermented soya beverage can also do the following:

- **Halt angiogenesis** Haelan helps cut off the blood supply to cancer cells.[27]

- **Promote apoptosis** In other words Haelan helps cancer cells die. In one study it reduced the anti-apoptosis gene expression BC12 on breast cancer cells twice as effectively as chemotherapy (doxorubicin – a drug which comes with the risk of leukaemia, heart failure, infertility, vomiting and mouth sores). It also *increased* the pro-apoptosis gene expression 500 per cent better than doxorubicin.[28]

- **Supercharge immunity 700 per cent**[29] Haelan has been shown to significantly boost the number of large white blood cells that digest cellular debris.

- **Treat 'treatment-resistant' cancers** Patients resistant to platinum chemotherapy (the standard treatment for ovarian cancer) have been shown to do remarkably well on Haelan; in one pilot trial it helped five ovarian cancer patients overcome a previous resistance to chemotherapy.[30]

▶

- **Reduce cachexia** Pronounced ka-kek-see-ah this is the wasting-away process that haunts end-stage cancer patients. According to Dr Allan Spreen, author of *Tomorrow's Cancer Cures TODAY*, cachexia is the major cause of death in cancer patients.[31] In a peer-reviewed multi-centre hospital study, Haelan was shown to reduce cachexia.[32]

- **Reduce circulating oestrogen levels** Haelan has been shown to significantly lower the oestrogens which damage cellular DNA and increase breast, ovarian and other hormone-driven cancers. Studies have shown an 81 per cent decrease in the 'bad oestrogens' for healthy women consuming this whole soya product.[33]

Hope for liver and pancreatic cancer?

While much of the research on Haelan is focused on hormonally driven cancers, anecdotal evidence suggests it benefits other types of cancer too.

Walter H. Wainright recently declared: 'Fermented soy is for the ugly cancers.' This bold statement starts to make sense when you sift through the research. A construction superintendent in his sixties who was diagnosed with terminal liver cancer started to take the Chinese soya-bean concentrate along with Venus flytrap, red clover, CoQ10, liquid oxygen and pycnogenol.[34] Seven months later the man was pronounced cancer-free. His doctor was gobsmacked; he did not know of any other survivors of the cancer (cholangiocarcinoma). There are also reports of long-term pancreatic cancer survivors who credit Haelan with their survival.

▶

Commenting on the product's success, Walter Wainright says: 'Conceivably, advanced liver and pancreatic cancer patients, who typically have no chance of survival using chemotherapy by itself, may increase their lifespan, improve the quality of their lives and possibly become cancer-free by using Haelan along with their chemotherapy treatments.'[35] Wainright also says: 'Haelan is especially effective in treating liver cancer because it improves liver function, knocks out carcinogens in the liver and supports regeneration of liver cells.' It also helps with eczema, parasites, hepatitis,[36] cirrhosis and wound healing, according to reports. Wainright's research has received recognition by the National Cancer Institute (USA) and he is currently collaborating with the Institute for Molecular Oncology in Recklinghausen, Germany.

Making it more palatable

The product information for Haelan acknowledges that 'sometimes taste is a problem for some consumers' and recommends adding ten drops of stevia per 113g dose. Mum initially had to brace herself for the daily dose: she'd take a deep breath, hold her nose and remind herself of the benefits. Six months on? It was a piece of cake – sort of. She is still ordering suitcases of the stuff and thinks this is one treatment she will take indefinitely.

Soya milk, however, is not fermented. In fact, it's highly processed. Dr Al Sears, a practising physician with extensive experience in the fields of complementary and natural healthcare, explains that making soya milk involves 'washing the beans in alkaline or boiling them in a petroleum-based solvent;

bleaching, deodorising and pumping them full of additives; heat-blasting and crushing them into flakes; and then mixing them with water to make "milk".'[37]

Still fancy that soya chai latte?

And there's another glaring problem with modern soya products. These days they're often genetically modified. 'I'm dead against anything GM and there's plenty of good reason for that,' says Patrick Holford. 'There's just so much we don't know about genetic modification.' Indeed, the reason we know so little about genetically modified food is because the manufactures won't allow it. As the *Scientific American* points out, the only tests approved are those that the manufacturers decide are 'friendly'.[38]

However, independent research from countries like Italy, Turkey and Denmark[39] has linked GM foods to infertility, weakened immune system, accelerated ageing, genetic problems with cholesterol, insulin control, cell signalling and protein formation, changes in the liver, kidney, spleen and gastrointestinal system and, more recently, cancer.[40]

Tasty Dairy and Soya Alternatives

From almond milk ice cream to raw truffle chocolate there is a mountain of options out there for the dairy- and soya-free consumer today. Alternative 'milks' now have their own dedicated supermarket aisles: hemp milk, rice milk, quinoa milk ... the choices are endless and the health benefits manifold. According to Christine O'Brien, editor of the monthly newsletter *Nutrition & Healing*, almond milk is 'absolutely packed' with nutrients: 'It's high in both protein and omega fatty acids, it's high in iron, calcium, potassium, magnesium and zinc, as well as the antioxidants vitamin A and vitamin E. All this without any cholesterol or saturated fat.'[41]

If you decide to buy your own non-dairy milk it pays to read labels. Some alternative 'milks' on the market often contain a host of less desirable ingredients including canola oil (which can cause macular degeneration), emulsifiers and E numbers. Then there's the issue of the plastic and aluminium-coated tetra packs that they typically come in. The answer? Make your own. 'It's so easy: just soak and blend!' says Natasha Corrett, UK-based vegetarian chef and co-author of *Honestly Healthy*. All you need to do is mix a cup of pre-soaked (overnight) almonds with 1 litre of water in a high-speed blender until smooth. Then, strain through a muslin cloth (or nut-milk bag).

Inspired by Natasha Corrett, I bought myself a nut-milk bag last year. To my surprise I found the homemade milk not only tasted creamier than store-bought alternatives, but it also seemed to blend more easily with hot drinks. I soon stopped feeling any kind of pangs for my morning latte and, in the course of writing this book, I have given up dairy (almost) entirely. Butter has been swapped for tahini, Asian recipes figure strongly in my repertoire and I have persuaded friends to occasionally meet at raw vegan restaurants (which appear to be popping up everywhere), rather than the usual high-street haunts. I have lost weight and no longer feel bloated after meals – enough of a motivation to keep my fridge milk-free. For now, my body tells me it's the right decision.

For her part, mum has finally got used to drinking oolong tea (a combination of black and green), she has perfected her olive oil mash and now cooks more Indian than Italian food. 'It means I'm eating a lot more immune-boosting spices like turmeric, galangal, ginger and coriander,' she says. Instead of relying on yoghurt to boost gut-friendly bacteria, mum now drinks kombucha (a fermented tea) daily.

If you're finding it tough to give up dairy, don't berate yourself for a lack of willpower; it might be as addictive as drugs: 'Dairy cheeses are a hard habit to break due to the opiate receptors they activate in our brains,' says integrative oncologist Dr Thomas Lodi. According to Dr Jo Esposito all mammals have morphine in their milk: 'It's there so babies calm down when they are breast-fed. Cow's milk has ten times the amount of morphine as human milk. Cheese is basically concentrated morphine.'[42]

So next time a craving kicks in, what can you reach for?

In the UK I've discovered Bessant and Drury's coconut milk ice cream (it beats Ben and Jerry's hands down) while in Australia my sister-in-law recently introduced me to Co-Yo, a brand of coconut yoghurt so delicious she calls it her desert island dessert. It's now available in the UK too. If you're craving creamy pasta, pine nuts and cashews can go a long way to making you forget about Parmesan, and if you were previously hooked on kefir, there are now plenty of coconut- and cashew-based alternatives. You might also want to stock up on 'raw' dairy-free chocolate for times of need. With no ingredients heated beyond 42 degrees the full health benefits of the chocolate are maintained (few people realise cocoa is one of the richest sources of magnesium, known as an anti-cancer powerhouse[43]). Mum will munch on a slice of raw chocolate when she's craving a treat – 'It feels much more like celebration than deprivation,' she says.

It's often remarked that when a family member gets cancer the whole tribe is moved to make healthy changes. It's certainly true of our family, all of whom are currently experimenting with varying degrees of lactose-free. I have almost completely cut it out (special occasions aside), my little brother has cut down and my younger sister, living in Paris and immersed in the world of gourmet food, likes the idea ... but is always looking for loopholes: she called me the other day, in the middle of making Tuscan bean soup. 'Now I just cook it with the Parmesan rind – does that count?' she said.

Being too puritanical is probably also carcinogenic.

CHAPTER 9

•

Getting in the O-zone

*'If ozone therapy were patentable, it would
be used in every physician's office and in
every hospital in the world.'*
Dr Horst Kief, prominent German physician

We all know how important oxygen is for our survival –
breath is life. But few people realise how vital it is for the
prevention of cancer, despite research dating back over seventy-
five years. In the 1930s Dr Otto Warburg, a Nobel Prize-winning
physician from Germany, discovered that low oxygen levels
were one of the key causes of cancer. He believed that cancer
cells are normal cells that have been forced to adjust to a low
oxygen environment in order to survive. Warburg explained his
findings in a presentation in 1966:[1] 'Cancer cells meet their
energy needs by fermentation, not oxidation. Thus, they are
dependent on glucose and a high oxygen environment is toxic
to them,'[2] he said. In other words, cancer cells love sugar (see
'Why Cancer Loves Sugar', overleaf) and hate oxygen.

Why Cancer Loves Sugar

It might be tempting to indulge in a cupcake when you're feeling tired and vulnerable, but if you've got cancer, you're playing with fire: 'We know that a cancer cell has ninety-six receptor sites for sugar. A normal cell has four,' says Dr Leigh Erin Connealy, in the film *CANCER is curable NOW*. Despite sugar being a well-known cancer accelerator, patients are rarely told to give up their favourite foods. In fact, at oncological centres across the globe, biscuits, ice cream and other sugar-laden snacks often feature on the menu.

Naturopath and clinical nutritionist David J. Getoff thinks it's unforgivable for a practitioner to be unaware of the sugar–cancer connection: 'Any physician that doesn't know cancer cells love sugar needs to immediately lose his or her licence and the reason is because they know that the way we find metastases around the body is with a PET scan,' he says. Before patients have a PET scan they are given an injection of radioactive sugar to make the cancer cells light up; this diagnostic tool *relies* on the fact that cancer cells love sugar: 'The cancer cells go, "Oh my favourite food! Thank you!" They gobble the sugar up, now the tumours are all radioactive and they glow on the PET scan,' explains Getoff.

Healthy cells transform into glucose-guzzling machines when they lose the ability to use oxygen effectively. Instead of being aerobic they become partially anaerobic and turn to fermentation as a way of producing energy. Dr Thomas Lodi, a leading integrative oncologist, explains why a fermentative state robs the body of energy: 'While a healthy cell will a grab a molecule of glucose, run it

▶

through its mitochondria with oxygen, produce thirty-eight energy packages that are called ATPs, cancer cells will grab that same molecule of glucose and produce only two ATPs – two energy packages. So cancer cells are nineteen times less efficient at energy production than healthy cells and to survive they need nineteen times more glucose.'

The link between fermentation and cancer is well documented. Decades ago two researchers at the National Cancer Institute discovered that the more aggressive a cancer was, the higher its glucose fermentation rate, and the slower-growing a cancer was, the lower its fermentation rate.[3] 'Studies looking at breast cancer biopsies show that the stage of the disease and how far it has metastasised correlates to the volume of insulin receptors,' says Dr Lodi. 'If that research were followed up, doctors really wouldn't need to do PET scans, since a biopsy would tell them how far the cancer had spread.'

Today you will find sugar in everything from toothpaste to tomato ketchup. To give you some idea of the dramatic rise in sugar consumption, in the US in 1822 the average person consumed 6.3 pounds a year, while in 1999, the average person consumed 107.7 pounds of sugar.[4] The sweet stuff has many disguises: look out for labels that include corn syrup, dextrose, maltose, glucose or fructose. And don't assume that organic, 'healthy' snacks are exempt from contamination – they're not. David Getoff reminds patients that alcohol and starch are also off the menu, if you want to stop feeding cancer cells their favourite food. 'So a no-starch diet means no potatoes, sweet potatoes, yams, corn or grains,' he clarifies. ▶

The ubiquity and addictiveness of sugar and starch are thought to be an underlying cause of not only cancer but also other life-threatening conditions like type-2 diabetes and heart disease.

So what's the answer? Fill your diet with whole, unprocessed foods, cut out artificial sweeteners, sodas and fruit juices and curb cravings by eating more protein or trying something sour. 'Incorporating fermented foods is a good first step for changing the body's craving for sweet foods,' says Donna Gates, nutritionist, lecturer and author of *The Body Ecology Diet*. 'Fermented foods are ideal for appetite and weight control, very alkaline and cleansing to the blood.' Of course, *eating* fermented food, regarded by many as having anti-cancer properties, will *not* fuel the fermentation process that is linked to cancer cells.

Cancer cells also tend to be more acidic, according to research.[5] Author and physician Dr Mark Sircus explains why: 'The lactic acid produced by fermentation lowers the cell pH (acid/alkaline balance). The cancer cells then begin to multiply unchecked.' So what causes the body to become oxygen deficient and acidic? Living in a polluted city, eating too many acid-forming foods (like dairy, sugar, bread, coffee and alcohol) and stress are three of the big ones. 'Stress will cause you to take shallow breaths,' explains New York-based cancer counsellor and researcher Dr Kelly Turner. 'After ten years of intense stress, you've got cells that have been starved of oxygen enough that their mitochondria might be damaged.' Dr Turner thinks we can learn a lot from babies: 'They take these beautiful belly breaths – they sleep a lot, they take naps, they're not working all day and they're moving,' she says.

Oxidative Therapies, Supersized Healing

Improving your breathing is certainly one way you can help keep cancer at bay (see box, below). But for those who truly want to get on top of their condition, simply getting more oxygen might not be enough. Many physicians believe *oxidative* therapies – including ozone therapy and hydrogen peroxide – are the real game-changers. 'Rather than simply sending more oxygen to cells, ozone works deep within the cells, stimulating mitochondria to use the oxygen that's already available,' explains medical journalist and health researcher Lee Euler, author of *Cancer Defeated!* Since the 1900s oxidative therapies have been used to treat a wide variety of conditions, from hepatitis and herpes[6] to diabetes and arteriosclerosis.[7] Much of the research has come out of Germany, Russia and Cuba, with the English-speaking world lagging woefully behind. But a number of pioneering doctors aim to change all that.

Simple Ways to Boost Your Oxygen Intake

From daily humming to dry brushing, there are many simple steps you can take to increase the oxygen levels in your body.

- **Start humming** Walking and humming dramatically increases oxygen intake, according to Marcus Freudenmann: 'The vibrations from humming soothe the nerves while helping to increase the flow of oxygen through the body,' he says. There's even a clinic in Denmark where patients walk through the garden humming and singing twice a day. 'They do it to ground their body, to flood it with free electrons and to oxygenate it,' says Freudenmann.

▶

- **Drink your greens** 'Green juice is the new Starbucks in celebrity circles – the only drink to be papped with,'[8] wrote one journalist in *The Times*. And mum is on trend: most days she makes herself a potent green cocktail, using a low-speed juicer and combining organic spinach leaves, broccoli sprouts, kale, wheatgrass and celery with a small apple or beetroot to sweeten the mix. According to Dr Thomas Lodi it's a great way to oxygenate your system: 'Chlorophyll [in green vegetables] improves oxygen transport throughout your body,' he says.

- **Breathe better** Learning to swap shallow breathing for deep breathing is one of the most important things you can do for health. In their book, *The Golden Ratio Lifestyle Diet*, Dr Robert Friedman and Mathew Cross suggest a breathing exercise, based on the divine Golden Ratio:[9] 'Upon awakening . . . inhale fully through your nose and into your abdomen to the count of three; then exhale to the count of five. Repeat this breathing pattern for at least eight cycles. Keep breathing slowly and deeply. As your breathing capacity improves, try inhaling to the count of five and exhaling to the count of eight. Go only as far as is comfortable for you. Now your blood is super-oxygenated and you're ready for your day.'

- **Blow bubbles** 'Not the kind that children play with,' says Dr Mark Sircus, 'but serious bubbles that one blows through a simple breathing retraining device.' Russian researchers recently developed the tool, the

▶

Breathslim, to aid asthma sufferers. But it's useful for cancer patients too: 'It really is quite nice to blow bubbles while increasing the oxygenation of your cells and tissues,' says Sircus.

- **Exercise** 'One of the best ways to oxygenate the body is by exercising,' says Dr Thomas Lodi, who encourages patients to do yoga. 'Yoga effectively facilitates the detoxification of body and mind by promoting circulation of blood and lymph fluid and by stimulating digestion,' he says. Going for a walk in nature is another good way of purifying your body, mind and spirit. It's something mum now does every day; when her busy mind turns to her to-do list, she takes a deep breath and focuses on her beautiful surroundings. On alternate days mum also jumps on a mini trampoline – another great way to oxygenate the blood[10] (see Chapter 7).

- **Give at-home oxygen a go** The low hum of mum's oxygen machine is often to be heard in the early evening. Sometimes my younger brother will be lounging around on her bed, keeping her company and waiting for his turn; sometimes it's just her and the greyhound – Dahling – poking her long nose in mum's masked face as she wobbles from side to side on her chi machine or bounces on the tramp. If you, like mum, decide to have oxygen therapy at home, a healthcare professional will work out with you how much oxygen you'll need and how long you'll need it for. But as general advice, California-based physician Dr Robert Jay Rowen says: 'Avoid a mask delivery at

▶

higher than 4 litres of oxygen per minute unless you are exercising.' Rowen has written extensively about EWOT – Exercise With Oxygen Therapy. 'Breathing 100 per cent oxygen *with* exercise ensures your body is creating the required levels of CO_2 to maintain balance in the body,' he explains.

- **Try dry brushing** Reports show that just five minutes of dry brushing can boost lymphatic drainage, stimulate the liver and oxygenate the blood by getting rid of dead skin cells and letting your skin breathe. 'Before I got the cancer I would literally *smother* my body in moisturiser, trying to make my skin soft,' says mum. 'But you know what? That's exactly what I was doing, I was *smothering* my pores.' Dry brushing quickly became part of mum's morning routine – it allowed her pores to open, so air could travel back and forth. 'Strangely enough, my skin doesn't seem to be any drier than before,' mum says.

From London to Los Angeles innovative physicians are witnessing stunning results thanks to oxidative therapies. Dr Robert Jay Rowen is one of them. 'I have been in ozone longer than anybody in North America. I think it's the ultimate anti-ageing therapy. I do it on a regular basis,' says the California-based physician. Dr Rowen regularly runs workshops on ozone therapy, hydrogen peroxide and ultraviolet blood irradiation and has educated hundreds of doctors around the world about their benefits.[11] 'I knew there had to be a better way to treat cancer,' he says. 'So I turned to studying combinations of oxidation therapy, which could be helpful in assisting deficiencies in the immune system and circulation in cancer patients. The goal was not to treat the cancer, but to treat the body of the patient to maximise its immune defences across the board.'

Taming Tumours

Dr Rowen has used oxidative therapies to treat a wide variety of conditions including asthma, heart disease and Lyme disease, but nowhere has he witnessed a more profound effect than with cancer. 'We've got one remission from a patient with terminal colon cancer, and I mean *terminal*,' he says. 'I didn't think he had a prayer. And he is now alive and well today with no trace of cancer.' The patient, 'SA', came to Dr Rowen aged seventy-six, with end-stage colon cancer and two metastatic tumours in his liver (11 and 9cm respectively). 'He looked like imminent death and had perhaps a few weeks to live at best,' says Rowen. Within four months of starting treatment, which included intravenous ozone and ultraviolet blood irradiation, SA's liver tumours had shrunk 85 per cent. This remarkable reduction was achieved without damaging healthy tissue or decimating the patient's defences. 'He is an Indian Swami, sort of an irascible type, and he didn't do everything I wanted him to do,' says Dr Rowen. 'He stubbornly refused to come in for every [twice weekly] appointment. None the less, after sixteen months, his liver tumours disappeared completely.' With the metastases gone, all that was left to tackle was SA's colon tumour, which was taken care of with surgery. Today, SA has no trace of cancer.

While Dr Rowen typically uses ultraviolet blood irradiation (UVBI) and intravenous ozone, other practitioners favour less well-known oxidative therapies: 'Our preference for ozone treatment here at the clinic is rectal insufflation,' says Dr Thomas Marshall-Manifold, a practitioner of biological medicine in Wimbledon, London. Others believe hyperbaric ozone therapy is best for cancer patients, while many practitioners around the world swear by hydrogen peroxide. 'It's incredibly cheap and very effective,' says British cancer expert and author Dr Patrick Kingsley. Among Kingsley's success stories was Edie Hubbard who was cured of end-stage breast cancer after she was given months to live (see Chapter 4).

It must be stressed, however, that oxidative therapies alone are rarely the answer. 'One of the problems we have is that somebody walks into the office and they say, "I want ozone, I've read it will cure my cancer,"' says Dr Marshall-Manifold, 'and you've got to say, "Well, it can help, but it's not a miracle."' However, when combined with other treatments, lifestyle changes, love, sunshine, nourishing foods and a connection to spirit, oxidative therapies can help bring cancer under control. This chapter looks at the most cutting-edge oxidative therapies and gives you some take-home tips for boosting your cellular oxygen levels (see page 177).

Ozone Therapy

Ever noticed the unusual smell after a storm? According to Nathaniel Altman, author of *The Oxygen Prescription: The Miracle of Oxidative Therapies*, it is a result of the small amounts of ozone in the air: 'Ozone is formed by the action of electrical discharges of oxygen, so it is often created by thunder and lightning,' he writes. Ozone is what makes the sky blue; it provides our planet with a protective layer from the sun's UV rays; and for almost a hundred years it has been used medicinally to treat a wide variety of diseases. The German army used ozone extensively during World War I to treat battle wounds and anaerobic infections, says Altman. Prior to that ozone gas was used to disinfect operating rooms in Switzerland. Today physicians around the world are using ozone to treat a wide spectrum of diseases including AIDS, asthma, cancerous tumours, cystitis, gangrene, herpes, rheuma-toid arthritis and Parkinson's disease.[12] 'Ozone is a powerful regulator of the immune system,' says Dr Dan Cullum, a leading integrative physician based in Oklahoma. 'This means that when the immune system is overactive – as in auto-immune disease – ozone will calm it down. Conversely, when the immune system is underactive as in cancer, AIDS and chronic infections, ozone will stimulate it.'

You can think of ozone as a supercharged oxygen molecule – O_3 rather than O_2. The addition of this extra atom makes ozone highly reactive and effective at helping the body to heal from a host of conditions, including heart disease. Experts believe that ozone oxidises the plaque in arteries, allowing the removal of the breakdown products, unclogging the blood vessels. When intro-duced into the bloodstream ozone triggers an avalanche of beneficial changes: it improves the exchange of oxygen in the blood, boosts circulation[13] and activates the immune system: 'Oxidative therapies induce your white blood cells to make tumour-killing properties,' explains Dr Rowen. 'All conventional research on the subject shows how increasing oxygen tension in tumours tames them.'

Mum started having intravenous ozone twice weekly follow-ing her diagnosis, alongside intravenous vitamins. (Many experts now believe that the body needs to be properly oxygenated for the vitamin C to work – see Chapter 4.)

But what does IV ozone involve? 'The patient sits in a chair and has from six to twelve ounces of blood removed into a sterilised bottle,' explains Dr Cullum. 'Then ozone is injected into the bottle and the bottle is gently shaken, allowing the red and white blood cells to take up the ozone. The ozonated blood is then returned to the body. The entire procedure takes about thirty to forty minutes.' This non-toxic treatment is said to increase the amount of oxygen in the blood by up to six times.[14]

But isn't ozone dangerous?

In sprawling metropolises like Sao Paulo and Mexico City ozone-laced smog is a major health hazard. In fact it's so destructive that it's even capable of corroding buildings, according to Altman. But the ozone that hangs over urban areas is very different from the kind you will find in a doctor's office: 'Medical ozone differs from atmospheric ozone in that it is pure and concentrated,' clarifies Marcus Freudenmann, producer of the hit documentary *CANCER is Curable NOW*. 'Atmospheric ozone is combined with nitrous oxide and sulphur oxide and is, therefore, dangerous. But many believe *medical ozone* to be the most promising, safe and generally efficacious treatment for major degenerative diseases,' he says. Dr Cullum believes that pure medical-grade ozone, when used along established medical guidelines, has an unparalleled safety record: 'Ozone is found naturally in the body. The white cells make it as part of the immune response,' he says. According to Dr Rowen oxidation therapies are 'almost completely non-toxic', while Dr Garry Gordon, co-founder of the American College for Advancement in Medicine (ACAM), also considers them 'entirely safe', but urges any practitioner planning to add ozone to their practice to take the necessary training.

An Ozone Colonic

Interestingly, the most harmless and economical way of delivering ozone is thought to be via the colon.[15] Dr Marshall-Manifold, who is based in Wimbledon, London, has been practising ozone therapy for over twenty-five years: 'I first saw ozone being used during my training in West Germany in the 1980s,' he says. 'It was being administered to a seventy-year-old woman with a breast tumour. The doctors were injecting ozone around the tumour – and her tumour was regressing.'

So why deliver ozone through the colon? 'It is a very efficient way of getting the ozone into the total system,' says Marshall-Manifold. 'That's why the French are so fond of suppositories; it's a useful way of delivering medication because the blood supply from the colon, through the portal vein, goes directly to the liver,' he explains. According to Nathanial Altman, 'rectal insufflation' – as it is known – has been around since the 1930s and is safe and effective. This is borne out by extensive research from Cuba and Italy showing its vast benefits[16] and demonstrating its low toxicity.[17] (In fact, Cuba is the only country in the world that offers ozone therapy on national insurance and they are responsible for much of the leading research.) A 2004 study found that intra-rectal applications of ozone reversed the toxicity caused by chemotherapy (cisplatin) and reduced kidney damage.[18]

So what does it involve?

'The day before treatment, patients have to take magnesium citrate salts at home,' says Marshall-Manifold. 'It liquefies everything, so they come in for their treatment with a totally clear colon.' Does it hurt? 'We use a very small tube and the [ozone] gas is seeped in, it's not *pumped* in,' Dr Marshall-Manifold explains reassuringly. 'It probably takes four to five minutes, then you leave the patient and let the ozone interact with the blood. The patient might feel a little bit windy or a little bit bloated afterwards, but that should only last about one or two hours. So the whole session lasts about half an hour.'

If you're a patient of Dr Cullum, expect to have a colonic irrigation prior to having ozone delivered up the unmentionable.

How often should you have it?

Dr Marshall-Manifold typically suggests weekly sessions for cancer patients, for a period of six weeks: 'If the markers are going down, you would step back [after four to six sessions] and let the body rest for a while, and then you might do three more sessions.' Like all the doctors I have interviewed for this book, Dr Marshall-Manifold stresses that there is no such thing a single standard protocol for patients. He builds programmes for his patients based on their laboratory results, nutritional profile and lifestyle. And his individualised approach is yielding results: just one of his success stories, a fifty-year-old woman with ovarian cancer, was successfully treated with a combination of rectal insufflations, vitamin B injections and superoxide dismutase (an enzyme that scavenges the harmful free radical, superoxide), along with vitamins A, D and C and selenium; a few weeks into her treatment the patient reported relief from her symptoms, and one month in her CA 125 (a marker for ovarian cancer) had gone from >500 KU/L (indicative of a residual tumour) to 18KU/L, which is well within the normal range.

Finding a practitioner who specialises in rectal insufflation is no mean feat; your search may well hit a bum note. If that's the case, you'll be pleased to know it's possible to have the treatment at home. Dr Rowen suggests purchasing your own ozone machine: 'With the help of a doctor familiar with ozone, you can most easily adapt it for your use for rectal insufflation,' he says.

One of my readers did just that. After trying rectal insufflation at a clinic, Vincent Crewe from Yorkshire decided it would be more cost-effective – and convenient – to purchase his own generator. He began self-administering the ozone in the comfort of his own home – sometimes rectally and other times through the skin (using a cupping device). 'I keep the ozone generator next to my infrared sauna in the guest bedroom. I'm sure visitors wondered what the hell was going on when they stayed – what with the large black oxygen cylinder and something that resembles Dr Who's TARDIS – but they never asked! One day I had the idea of combining the treatments, since I knew the heat would keep my pores wide open while I funnelled the ozone in.' Being the innovative individual that he is, Vincent drilled a small hole in the side of the sauna cabinet, just big enough to insert the ozone output tube, and attached a special ozone funnel to it. 'I can then funnel the ozone directly over the spot where the tumour was removed. I do this for the last twenty minutes of each sauna session,' he says. (See Chapter 12 for more on Vincent's healing journey.)

Ultraviolet Blood Irradiation (UVBI)

By the early 1940s UVBI was being used in several American hospitals, and by 1949 *Time* magazine was calling it the wave of the future.[19] In this therapy a small amount of blood is withdrawn from the patient, exposed to UV light then returned to the body. The process has been shown to improve oxygenation of tissues, stimulate the immune system and lead to increased tolerance of conventional cancer treatments. In one study, patients who had suffered a drop in red blood cell counts due to chemotherapy had 200ml of blood removed, irradiated and reintroduced into the body. The red blood cell counts returned to normal.[20] Dr Jay Rowen has been seeing improvements in cancer patients using a combination of UVBI and ozone. He typically suggests twice weekly appointments, gradually tapering the sessions down if the patients start to improve.

We've been schooled to believe UV is harmful, but it's not the whole story. 'For eons nature has utilised the sun's ultraviolet energy as a cleansing agent for the earth,' explains Dr Rowen. 'Obviously, if you get an excess of ultraviolet light on your skin, you get a burn. But you need some ultraviolet light.' Health researcher Lee Euler agrees: 'The treatment [UVBI] is absolutely completely safe and has *no* side effects.'

However, the promising treatment, like so many others, was eclipsed by the introduction of antibiotics. 'UVBI was almost completely set aside, even though a number of diseases, including hepatitis, streptococcal toxemia and viral pneumonia, actually responded better to UVBI therapy than to antibiotics and vaccines,' says Dr Jonathan Wright, a renowned authority on alternative medicine and medical director of Tahoma Clinic in Seattle. 'It's well past time medicine goes "back to the future" and starts using this long-ago-proven therapy.'

Hydrogen Peroxide

It's been written about in respected, peer-reviewed medical journals since 1888.[21] Over 6100 articles in European scientific literature have vouched for the effectiveness of this simple therapy[22] and evidence suggests that around 15,000 European practitioners have treated over 10 million patients with it.[23] Many have seen first-hand end-stage cancer patients come back from the brink within weeks of starting the inexpensive protocol.

Although it may sound like a formidable substance, hydrogen peroxide is actually produced by every cell in your body. 'It's abundant in mother's milk, it's abundant in rain, it's ubiquitous throughout nature, so it's a very fundamental molecule,' says Dr Thomas Lodi. Interestingly, healing springs around the world, including Fatima in Portugal, Lourdes in France and the Shrine of St Anne in Canada, have been found to contain hydrogen peroxide.[24]

Hydrogen peroxide (H_2O_2) is essentially water (H_2O) with an extra oxygen atom attached. Your own white blood cells make some hydrogen peroxide, as a way of killing invading 'nasties' such as fungi, viruses or cancer. 'When you use it in a specific concentration it stimulates the whole oxidative system, which is the way you kill off foreign invasions including abnormal cells like cancer,' explains Dr Lodi.

In 2001 a group of researchers from the Department of Life Sciences at Nottingham Trent University in England injected hydrogen peroxide solutions into solid tumours in mice. They concluded that hydrogen peroxide was a potent agent: 'Hydrogen peroxide can act as an anti-cancer drug with two distinct advantages over conventional therapeutic agents: it produces minimal short- and long-term side effects and is relatively cheap and cost-effective.'[25]

Is it safe?

When properly administered hydrogen peroxide has been shown in countless studies to be non-toxic. However, if you're going to take it orally you should be under medical supervision. Dr Patrick Kingsley warns that it can sometimes upset a person's stomach. For that reason, he doesn't personally recommend it, although he says: 'I happen to know there are millions of people throughout the world, who swear by the protocol.' Although mum decided against IV H_2O_2 in the end, as the travel time involved ran counter to the promise she had made to put joy back on the agenda (see Chapter 3), many patients have gone the distance.

For decades Dr Patrick Kingsley treated thousands of patients with intravenous vitamins, minerals and hydrogen peroxide at his clinic in the English Midlands. 'Many patients came from long distances, so sometimes hydrogen peroxide was a better option than vitamin C since you only needed an hour and a half,' he says, adding that vitamin C could sometimes take up to three hours. 'I would give it [IV H_2O_2] to patients as often as possible and very effective it was indeed.'

A healing hot tub?

While hydrogen peroxide is typically administered intravenously, there are other ways of getting it in. Some integrative practitioners suggest adding four cups of 35 per cent H_2O_2 to the bath[26] as a way of detoxing (something mum does regularly); others recommend a few drops of H_2O_2 in a vaporiser or nebuliser to deal with breathing problems. 'We have been using H_2O_2 in a nebuliser for any type of respiratory disease, either acute or chronic,' says Dr Robert L. White, a leading proponent of oxidative therapies.

One of my readers from Australia, Lance Hand, has been inhaling hydrogen peroxide since his diagnosis of prostate cancer. 'You simply buy a nasal-spray bottle and fill it with 3 per cent food-grade hydrogen peroxide, then squirt it down your throat while inhaling sharply. The spray goes into the lungs and is absorbed into the bloodstream and, of course, misses the stomach. I also brush my teeth with it and wash the veggies with it to clear off any fungus or bacteria.'

Which Hydrogen Peroxide Do I Use?

Important: hydrogen peroxide comes in many strengths. For general purposes – to clean your veggies, brush your teeth or use in an inhaler – a 3 per cent solution is recommended. However, the much more powerful (and potentially toxic) food-grade 35 per cent hydrogen peroxide can be diluted by carefully adding to still water. Mum uses this type in her bath.

Speaking to a qualified practitioner on these matters is absolutely to be advised. Yet sadly, there is a dearth of practitioners schooled on the subject of hydrogen peroxide. 'There are very few people in the country who do hydrogen peroxide and that's a great shame,' says Kingsley. So why don't more physicians offer this treatment? 'The real problem with peroxide is that it won't bring in money,' writes George Borell in *The Peroxide Story*. 'It is a natural substance and therefore can't be patented.

There is really nothing the drug companies can do about it except scare people into thinking that it is bad for them.'

Some believe hydrogen peroxide represents *the* biggest threat to the trillion-dollar earnings of the pharmaceutical companies – a bottle of food-grade H_2O_2 can be bought for around £1 from a chemist. Small wonder, then, that it's often written off as dangerous. Dr Keith Scott-Mumby is weary of the criticisms. In *Cancer Research Secrets* he writes: 'There have been claims it is dangerous and one doctor, I know, was charged with murder because a cancer patient died while having peroxide treatment. In fact, the patient died of his cancer, but that inconvenient truth doesn't stop the bigots of orthodoxy from attacking anything they hate,' he says. 'You will notice that no doctor gets charged with murder for administering deadly chemical cocktails and brutal radiation, or performing mutilating surgery. They always blame the cancer and say the patient died of that "despite everything we could do to save them".'

When properly administered hydrogen peroxide, UVBI and ozone will do no harm – one of the central tenets of the oft-quoted Hippocratic Oath (the oath historically taken by physicians). But will it work for everyone? That's another matter entirely. As with any cancer treatment, alternative or conventional, there are no guarantees. What works for one person will not necessarily work for the next, and one man's salvation can be another man's waste of time. That said we *all* need oxygen, so it stands to reason if there *are* ways of filling our tanks with more of this life force – whether through oxidative therapies, daily exercise, humming or body brushing – we'd be wise to take heed. Remember, cancer hates oxygen; life loves it.

CHAPTER 10

●

Low-dose Chemotherapy and Life-saving Tests

'If you're going to go down the chemotherapy route, go down it gently.'
Dr Thomas Lodi, integrative oncologist

What if I told you there was a test that could detect cancer four to six years earlier than current methods – a sophisticated technique that was 200 times more accurate than a PET scan *and* infinitely safer? Imagine if people could closely monitor their health and make necessary adjustments, so cancer became preventable, rather than inevitable. One in two people will be diagnosed with cancer in their lifetime according to current statistics.[1] Imagine the millions of lives that might be saved if cancer was picked up in micrograms, rather than at the stage of metastasis?

What if I also told you there was a way of determining which treatments – both alternative and conventional – would work best for your cancer; and all it took was a blood test or tissue sample? Imagine the deaths that might be avoided if oncologists were able to choose the 'right' chemotherapy from the start, rather than playing Russian roulette? What if this bespoke chemotherapy could also be administered at very low doses in a targeted way, so the patient was spared the indignity of hair loss, diarrhoea or worse?

This isn't science fiction, or a far-off distant reality. These groundbreaking tests and techniques are available right now. 'Cancer could become a controllable disease if my technique, the Tumour Marker Combination Assay, was made widely available,' says Dr Tsuneo Kobayashi, medical maverick and inventor of the innovative marker test. 'I believe it could save seven million people every year.'

In a world where new drugs are considered a triumph if they promise to extend life by a few short weeks, Dr Kobayashi's words sound slightly fantastical. But after successfully treating thousands of end-stage cancer patients over the past thirty years, and with the American Cancer Institute banging at his door, the sixty-nine-year-old physician has every right to speak plainly about the value of his work.

'He is an unrecognised hero,' says Dr Thomas Lodi, integrative oncologist and founder of An Oasis of Healing centre in Arizona. 'His Tumour Marker Combination Assay (TMCA) has a range of one through to five, one being zero cancer and five being one gram of cancer – the level when it is usually detectable.' Dr Garry Gordon, co-founder of the American College for Advancement in Medicine (ACAM) and another heavyweight in the world of holistic medicine, is similarly enthusiastic about Dr Kobayashi's work: 'He is a giant in the overall picture of cancer detection and treatment,' he says. 'He is a molecular biologist MD, who became a pathologist, who became an oncologist ... so there isn't anybody who can challenge his credentials. He's the real thing.'

Beyond Biopsies

In the 1980s the National Cancer Institute (NCI) in the USA put Kobayashi's marker system to the test. In one double-blind study, the Institute sent Kobayashi 360 blood samples consisting of forty early-stage colon cancer patients, thirty benign colon cancer patients and fifty healthy control subjects. Using his TMCA technique Kobayashi was able to correctly identify the presence of cancer in 87.5 per cent of the samples.

Conventional blood marker tests, on the other hand, can be extremely imprecise. Less than 25 per cent of patients with early stage colon cancer show an elevated CEA level.[2] Molecular oncologist Dr Papasotiriou believes conventional markers provide little benefit: 'CA 125 [the marker for ovarian cancer] is elevated in less than 30 per cent of patients; that means for 70 per cent it will be useless for diagnostic purposes,' he says. (However, if the patient *does* have an elevated CA 125 at the time of diagnosis – as mum did – the test can be used to monitor whether the treatment is working and whether there has been a relapse of disease, according to Dr Papasotiriou.)

Since conventional marker tests are unreliable, cancer patients are usually required to have an additional X-ray scan (CT or PET scan) and biopsy to confirm the presence of malignant cells. These procedures are not only expensive – they're dangerous. 'When you perform a biopsy on a cancerous tumour, it's not a question of whether you're causing cancer cells to spread: you *are*,'[3] says Dr Lodi. A PET scan delivers as much harmful radiation as a head, chest, abdomen, pelvis and bone scan combined, and recent research suggests that CT scans may contribute to around 29,000 new cancer cases every year.[4] But Dr Kobayashi's invention could render these standard screening tools obsolete.

Dr Kobayashi's Top Tips

Seven ways to keep cancer at bay – from Japan's medical maverick:

▶

- Follow a macrobiotic diet: think brown rice, sea vegetables, miso soup and balancing yin and yang.

- Live your life free of bitterness and full of delight.

- Give up dairy (see Chapter 8).

- Reduce your exposure to diagnostic radiation.

- Avoid additives, especially aspartame.

- Steer clear of cold food and beverages. 'Ingesting cold beverages can lead to latent infections in the intestinal tract,' says Dr Kobayashi. 'This, in turn, reduces intestinal immunity and can lead to cancer.'

- Avoid eating charred meat and fish. (To make your next BBQ less carcinogenic try marinating meat first. Researchers from Kansas State University found that when you add ginger root, rosemary and turmeric to meat before cooking at high temperatures, carcinogenic by-products[5] were reduced by as much as 87 per cent.)

Measuring Cancer in Micrograms

In the last twenty years, out of the 20,000 people who have taken Dr Kobayashi's test only three (all healthy teenagers) have received a reading of 'tumour stage I' – i.e. zero cancer. The majority of people – 60 per cent of those he has tested – are at stage III, meaning they have micrograms to milligrams of cancer in their bodies. 'Dr Kobayashi has got to a point now where if someone is at stage III he can tell them, 'This *will* become a colon cancer' or 'This *will* become an ovarian cancer'. His stage III is about two and a half to three years away from being clinically manifest,' says Dr Lodi. However, with his lifestyle advice and treatments Kobayashi can radically reduce a person's risk. A 'stage-III' patient, for example, might be advised to cut out dairy, avoid foods with chemical additives like aspartame and follow a macrobiotic way of eating. Dr Kobayashi might also recommend a course of Chinese herbs, acupuncture or a week of fasting.

But how effective are these simple lifestyle changes? The rebel oncologist believes his cancer-prevention programme is 99 per cent successful. He has kept 10,000 patients cancer-free over a ten-year period thanks to regular TMCA testing and individualised advice. With the epidemic rates of stomach cancer in Japan,[6] it's safe to assume that some of Dr Kobayashi's 10,000 might have otherwise developed the disease. But due to his expert advice, no one who followed his programme got cancer.

It takes seven years for a tumour to get big enough to be a 'lump or bump' according to Dr Garry Gordon. But if you used Dr Kobayashi's early-detection method, you would have time to make the necessary diet and lifestyle changes and avoid that eventuality. However, not everyone is willing to make the effort – as Dr Thomas Lodi discovered. He recalls meeting one woman at Dr Kobayashi's clinic in Japan who was found to be at 'stage III'. 'Two and a half years later I happened to be back there and I thought I recognised her in the waiting room,' he says. 'I asked Dr Kobayashi whether it was the same woman and he said, "Yes, she has breast cancer now." She had ignored his advice.'

When a late-stage cancer patient shows up in a conventional oncologist's office, the doctor will often talk about 'hitting the tumour hard' and 'throwing everything at it': the thinking goes that an 'aggressive' cancer warrants an 'aggressive' treatment. The problem with this approach, however, is that the physician is in a race against time to kill the cancer before the chemotherapy kills the patient. In an investigation of 600 case studies of cancer patients who died within thirty days of treatment, researchers discovered that 25 per cent of those deaths were directly caused or hastened by chemotherapy.[7] Dr Kobayashi, however, takes a very different approach to treating cancer.

'Delinquent', Not 'Malignant' Cells

'Western doctors believe cancer cells are malignant, but this is thoroughly wrong, because cancer cells are really like delinquent teenage boys,' asserts Dr Kobayashi. He believes cancer cells are neglected cells – they may have been malnourished or exposed to toxic substances – and what they really need is love and nutrients in order to heal. Melding Western and Eastern methods, Dr Kobayashi typically treats patients with a combination of modalities including hyperthermia, low-dose chemotherapy, high-dose vitamin C and other immune-boosting treatments. With this rigorous holistic programme, Dr Kobayashi believes he can send some 70 per cent of all his cancer patients into remission, even if they are in the last stage of the disease.[8] Sceptics might pounce on such a bold assertion, but Kobayashi has no shortage of patient success stories. Over the last thirty years he has treated over 6000 mid- to late-stage cancer patients with an average life span after treatment of seven years. In comparison, overall survival rates in the US are just 2.1 per cent over a five-year period for stage-4 adult cancer patients.[9]

Although patients don't *have* to travel to Japan for the test, the cost and complication of sending it make a long-haul flight seem like a breeze: 'If we send it to Japan it has to go through customs and it needs to have so much dry ice that it can cost you $600 in shipping fees alone,' says Gordon. 'Instead, I suggest my patients have an ultra-sensitive HCG urine test and PHI blood test, available through the American Metabolic Laboratories in Florida. If those tests find there is no cancer, there *is* no serious cancer in the body [see page 204].'

Early Detection – Can You Put A Price On It?

The billions poured into cancer research might be missing the main target. The National Cancer Institute spent just 8 per cent of its 2007 budget (less than $400 million) on detection. Likewise, the pharmaceutical industry spends around $8 billion annually on drug development for late-stage treatment,[10] despite the many more lives that would be saved if the cancer were caught in the early stages. Colon cancer, for example, has a 91 per cent five-year survival rate when diagnosed early, compared to an 11 per cent survival rate for late-stage colon cancer.[11]

Prevention seems to be the winning ticket, but those in positions of power aren't keeping their eye on the game. A few years ago Dr Garry Gordon handed all the research papers on Dr Kobayashi to a (former) head of the White House commission on alternative approaches to curing cancer. The result? 'He thanked me effusively and promptly managed to lose or misplace the file,' says Dr Gordon.

Dr Lodi and Low-dose Chemotherapy

Dr Thomas Lodi believes cancer is not a disease. 'Cancer is the body's extraordinary effort to keep you alive,' he says. Prior to attending medical school, Dr Lodi worked as a clinical psychologist – an experience which no doubt informed his open mind to medicine. For the first ten years of his medical career, Lodi worked as an internal medicine specialist, urgent-care physician and in the ICU and CCU departments of various hospitals. But after using conventional modalities for a decade Dr Lodi came to the clear conclusion that they 'didn't work'.

This epiphany led him on a quest around Japan, Europe and Mexico to discover more effective and less toxic therapies. For the last twelve years Dr Lodi has been putting his extensive training and experience into practice at his centre – An Oasis of Healing – where visitors are treated with a combination of oxidative therapies, high-dose vitamin C, colon cleansing and organ detoxification, as well as low-dose chemotherapy. Dr Lodi refers to chemo as a 'cytotoxic poison that kills cells'. So why use it at all? 'If the cancer is widespread or causing damage or disruption to a vital function like breathing, bowel movement or eating, we need to move fast and this is the most rapid way to do it,' says Dr Lodi. 'But if you're going to do it, do it gently.'

Most of us today are familiar with the effects of chemotherapy. We have all seen colleagues, friends and loved ones lose their hair, appetite and joie de vivre in the 'battle' against cancer. Chemotherapy targets rapidly dividing cells, which include not only cancer cells, but also the fast-replicating hair follicles and stomach cells – which explains why chemo can leave people feeling like they have a perpetual hangover.[12] But with Dr Lodi's low-dose chemotherapy the effects are far milder: 'You don't see the major side effects like hair loss,' says Dr Lodi. 'In my experience one out of twenty people experience nausea and, out of those, one out of ten will actually vomit. It's not the major event that it is with conventional chemo, which in my opinion is a horror, a nightmare – it violates all of nature's laws.'

Renutrifying the body

Cancer is the consequence of an overly toxic body, according to Dr Lodi. So when a patient arrives at An Oasis of Healing, they are given a combination of immune-boosting foods and therapies including vegetable juices, intravenous vitamin C, ozone and infrared saunas. Unless the tumour is impacting a vital function, Dr Lodi advises patients to spend two weeks on his detoxification programme before commencing low-dose chemo-therapy. But not all patients are *patient*: 'The problem is most people come here and say, "I have four weeks – fix me",' he says.

The Trojan horse treatment

The 'gentle' form of chemotherapy that Dr Lodi (and a growing band of clued-up oncologists) uses has come to be known as insulin-potentiated targeted low-dose therapy, or IPT. Fifteen years ago, Dr James Forsythe, founder of the Century Wellness Clinic in Nevada and author of *Take Control of Your Cancer*, switched to a more humane way of delivering chemotherapy after witnessing 'every horrible type of toxicity imaginable' thanks to conventional treatment. So how does it work? 'The theory behind the mechanism of IPT is based on the fact that cancer cells have many more insulin receptors on the cell surface than all the other cells in the body,' explains Dr Forsythe (see 'Why Cancer Loves Sugar', page 174). Therefore, small amounts of insulin trick the cancer cell into welcoming the chemotherapy, and lower doses – typically 10 per cent of the normal chemotherapy dose – are required. Ultimately, the insulin works like a Trojan horse to sneak the drug into the cancer cells. 'It's kind of a rational approach to poisoning someone, and it works,' says Dr Lodi.

Eeny, Meeny Miny, Che-mo

Choosing the *right* chemotherapy is just as important as using a low dose: 'To determine that everyone with a particular type of cancer should be given the same drug is like saying the average shoe size is nine, so that's the only size we'll make,' says Dr Lodi, who will often take a biopsy of the patient's tumour and send it to a lab: Rational Therapeutics in Long Beach, California. Run by Dr Robert Nagourney, the lab tests different drugs on the tumour and determines which work best. 'Once the right agent is identified I can be assured that any spread from the biopsy will be nipped in the bud. It's the only time I will do a biopsy on a patient.' The process takes five days.

Dr Nagourney's website is filled with testimonials from patients who owe their life to his sophisticated tests. When Elizabeth Panke was diagnosed with an extremely aggressive form of ovarian cancer in 1999 she tried chemotherapy. But after the second round of chemotherapy failed, she was given months to live. 'Rational Therapeutics exposed my tumour cells to chemotherapy drugs and observed which drugs actually killed my tumour cells ... Based on their recommendations, I immediately received treatment. Following six cycles of this chemotherapy, I had no evidence of tumour by CT scan, by PET scan, by ultrasound and by physical exam. Today, over ten years later, I can confidently say that I am cured of recurrent metastatic ovarian cancer!'[13]

Notwithstanding the evident benefit of Rational Therapeutics, the test has limitations. 'If cancer tissue is in the brain, lungs, liver, bones or deep in the pancreatic tissues, removing a sufficient amount of tissue for testing is not only difficult and risky to the patient's health, but may require a major surgical procedure,' says Dr Forsythe. The test also fails to look at the natural, non-toxic substances that will work best for the patient.

Testing, Testing ... One, Two, Three

Here are some important tests you might not know about.

Test your metal

On the recommendation of a holistic dentist in Harley Street, mum had a blood test to check her sensitivity to

▶

heavy metals. While a hair sample will measure the levels of metals in a patient's body, the MELISA test (Memory Lymphocyte ImmunoStimulation Assay) looks at whether the individual is allergic to those metals.

'This is very different to the "normal" allergic reaction you get from dust mites or grass pollen,' emphasises Olaf Beckord, director of the InVitaLab where mum had the test. 'It is, in fact, an inflammatory reaction which causes oxidative stress and may lead to cancer.' Scary stuff when you consider that up to 30 million Americans have metal allergies.[14]

Mum's MELISA test confirmed her deepest fear: she was allergic to gold – along with palladium, gallium, indium, copper, beryllium and nickel. 'To be allergic to seven metals is quite a lot; most people are only allergic to one or two,' says holistic dentist Dr Goran Stojanovic, from the Ella clinic on Harley Street. 'It means getting rid of any metals, especially in the mouth, needs to be a top priority for your mum.' Mercury fillings and root canals are the obvious culprits for metal contamination (see Chapter 6), but cosmetics, antiperspirant deodorants, pacemakers, jewellery and silicone breast implants should not be overlooked.

The hippie test kit

Cancer survivor, author and holistic practitioner Paul Winter has devised an alternative cancer test kit which contains vials imprinted with the 'energy signature' of twelve potent cancer treatments: 714x, Beta Glucan, Cantron, Cesium Chloride, Emulsified Vitamin A, Ellagic Acid, Essiac Tea, Hydrazine Sulphate, Laetrile, MGN-3, Paw Paw and Protocel.

▶

The kit relies on the principles of muscle testing, often used by chiropractors and kinesiologists. It proposes that every food or medicine has a unique energy signature and that our bodies respond to this energy signature in measurable ways. According to naturopath and clinical nutritionist David J. Getoff, when properly learned and correctly practised muscle testing 'may be the single most valuable method in existence for gathering information about a patient or client'. Alternative cancer treatments are, for the most part, tough to get hold of and hard on the wallet. The beauty of Winter's test kit is that it is affordable. You can purchase the test kit for $48 – a mere snip compared to the $800 it would cost to buy even tiny amounts of the listed treatments.

Early cancer detection – Stateside

American Metabolic Laboratories offers a specific panel of cancer tests – the 'CA-Profile'. Dr Garry Gordon recommends two in particular: HCG and PHI.

Better known as the pregnancy hormone, HCG (human chorionic gonadotropin) has been noted as a cancer marker since the 1950s, when Dr Manuel Navarro developed the eponymous 'Navarro urine test' after discovering HCG present in all types of cancers. American Metabolic Laboratories takes Navarro's test one step further, offering detection of the hormone at extremely low levels. Dr Gordon also recommends the PHI test (phosphohexose isomerase enzyme), which alerts you to the level of anaerobic metabolism going on in your body. 'Cancer only starts in cells that are anaerobic – cells that don't require oxygen to survive,' he says (see Chapter 9).

Mum Goes to Germany

Shortly after her diagnosis mum heard about a German laboratory called Biofocus. The laboratory, located just outside Dusseldorf, is at the forefront of 'molecular oncology' – an emerging field, which focuses on cancer detection and analysis at minute molecular levels. The lab also offers chemo-resistance testing and, to mum's excitement, 'alternative agent' testing.

So how does the test work? Using a sample of the patient's blood, the scientists look for what are called circulating tumour cells (CTCs). 'We analyse the genetic properties of these tumour cells and from this we can determine how effective the various treatments will be,' says Dr Lothar Prix, a molecular biologist from Biofocus.

Mum was eager to have the test done; she had, thus far, relied on research and intuition to guide her choice of alternative therapies, but was there a more fool-proof method? She was deeply curious, but she didn't feel strong enough, following her hysterectomy to travel to Germany. (While most patients ship their blood to the lab, it can be a logistical nightmare for those living as far away as Australia: samples must arrive at the Biofocus lab within forty-eight hours, and the flight alone is roughly twenty-two.) But with both her daughters living in Europe, it was only a matter of time before mum got itchy feet. So more than a year after her diagnosis, mum and I found ourselves on a train to the city of Recklinghausen, home to the famous laboratory.

Meeting Dr Prix

According to her last CA-125 blood test mum was cancer-free, but this molecular, highly sophisticated analysis brought a whole new meaning to the term 'all clear' and she couldn't help worrying what it would reveal. But the molecular biologist's calm, matter-of-fact way of speaking sent catastrophic fears packing and switched our rational brains back on. While a no-nonsense nurse took mum's blood – as if she was taking her temperature – I took the opportunity to quiz Dr Prix about molecular oncology. Something I couldn't get to grips with was how the test worked when we *all* have cancer cells in our bodies. The body produces cancer cells every day, as part of its normal metabolic process. That being the case, how could Dr Prix tell who *had* cancer and who didn't?

'Our research shows that normal individuals – without a history of cancer – have significantly lower levels of the genetic cancer markers,' Dr Prix explained. Between the years 2006 and 2007 researchers at Biofocus compared the blood samples of 'healthy' patients to those of stage-3 and 4 cancer patients. In 5 per cent of non-cancer patients, at least one genetic marker showed up abnormally. In contrast, 80 per cent of cancer patients showed at least one 'upregulated' marker. 'The more genetic markers we find, the more certain we can be that the cells we identify are really tumour cells,' says Dr Prix, adding that the tests are primarily for individuals who have been diagnosed with cancer and want to choose the best treatment.

High-dose vitamin C, Graviola, Laetrile, Haelan and hyperthermia are just some of the well-established alternative treatments Biofocus tests against. The lab also offers a 'Natural Killer Cell Test' which reveals how well a patient's immune system is working and uncovers the best natural substances to boost the body's defences. For this particular test only the patient's immune cells are required – no cancer cells.

If the alternative agent test came back with a blank page it would mean mum had no cancer cells to test against, and that her treatment plan was watertight. But the universe had other plans – and it seems we had other avenues to explore. Two and a half weeks after our visit to Germany mum received an email with her results. While three out of the four tumour markers were negative, one was *very slightly* raised. ERBB2 is linked to a few different types of cancers, including uterine cancer. Mum was gutted – at least initially. When I called her a few minutes after seeing the results she was deflated and confused. But after a closer look she rallied. The results showed that her immune system was super strong (operating at 27 out of a possible score of 30) and none of the other cancer markers was raised.

When I finally got hold of Dr Prix the following Monday, our worst fears were allayed. 'All other markers are negative and only ERBB2 is slightly elevated, so this is very borderline,' he said reassuringly. 'It's a very weak positive.' He also answered my questions about the recommended alternative treatments and advised me on where to get hold of them. The test revealed that the most beneficial treatment for mum at this point was a fermented soya therapy called Haelan – something we had never heard of (see Chapter 8).

Poor Dr Prix was confronted by my anxious phone call only an hour after he'd returned from his summer holiday; being a journalist I assume it's my God-given right to cold call experts and demand answers. But many who take these genetic tests can be left marooned, without a clue as to what to do with their results. Janet Mears, one of my blog subscribers from Perth, Australia, had her cancer cells genetically analysed with the Research Genetic Cancer Centre (RGCC) in Greece, another top laboratory. She recently contacted me to share her experience: 'I think some of the results concerning the gene factors would be useful if you had the right doctor. I showed them to a local oncologist and his first remark was, "That must have cost you a bit!" Then he threw it aside without looking at it. My German doctors gave me a treatment plan to go home with which included taking low-dose chemo tablets daily, but the oncologists here will not prescribe them ... I have been laughed at when I mentioned alternatives; they even say vitamin C is unproven!'

So how important is it to have a doctor fluent in molecular oncology and conversant in natural treatments? 'It's extremely important,' says Dr Papasotiriou from RGCC. 'We realised this very early on and that's why we are familiarising as many physicians as we can – through webinars, conferences and by contacting them directly. We also have an area on our website where patients and physicians can ask questions and request a Skype meeting with us,' he says.

Tomorrow's Early Detection

In May 2012, American teen Jack Andraka won the world's largest high-school science competition[15] for creating a way to test for pancreatic cancer: a disease for which no early detection method is currently available. At the age of fifteen, Andraka developed a test that is 168 times faster, 400 times more sensitive and 100 times more selective than the tests currently available. 'Most importantly, the test can diagnose pancreatic cancer at an early stage, before it spreads,' says Lee Euler, author and publisher of the highly acclaimed newsletter *Cancer Defeated!* 'Pancreatic cancer has traditionally been tough to diagnose . . . the current blood test isn't effective till patients are in the advanced stages of the disease, when the game is just about over.'

Jack Andraka came up with this potentially life-saving test using basic materials. He simply bought some diabetic test paper and a $50 electrical test meter from the local hardware store to create his innovative dipstick sensor test. Andraka says his test can be used for early diagnosis of lung and ovarian cancers as well. At the time of writing,

▶

multiple drug companies are in hot pursuit of this young science star, desperate to license or commercialise his test. Watch this space.

A Brighter Future

Dr Papasotiriou is clearly keen to raise awareness about the benefits of molecular oncology. He likens the genetic tests offered at RGCC to bespoke clinical trials: 'We have taken the same technologies used by the [R&D section] of pharmaceutical companies to identify, validate and assess candidate drugs and we simply apply them to each individual,' he says. 'The reason we do this, is that cancer is not one homogenous stable disease.'

If cancer could be picked up before it becomes a visible lump imagine how much easier it would be to treat? Dr Garry Gordon believes this is the area we need to focus on: 'It's only when people fail a test that they're going to spend money, change their diet, give up the sugar, start to walk, stop the smoking – nobody is going to do these things until they have a problem.'

We all like to believe we're immortal. We all believe that car accidents, heart attacks and chronic disease happen to other people – until they happen to us. This happy delusion allows us to continue life at a relentless pace until everything comes crashing down. That's when the second delusion kicks in: the belief that a doctor will cure us.

'Only *you* can do the dance that's required for the body to heal – all we can do is teach you,' says Dr Lodi. 'At our healing centre we have a library of books and a whole curriculum that we teach patients. But when they leave here, if they don't have a passion for reading and learning, they're going to return to old habits and get back to old tapes – old ways of thinking.'

Striking the right balance and staying healthy is something all of us struggle with. Life gets in the way and our best intentions crumble in the face of celebrations, stress and a drive for success. But if you don't make time to look after your health, as the saying goes, sooner or later you'll have to make time for illness. So if having a regular blood test is going to keep you on track, be sure to book that appointment. If you're like mum – who has read more health books than Gwyneth Paltrow has had green juices – then maybe that's all you need to stay motivated.

A few weeks after returning from Germany mum saw Val Allen, her naturopath, homeopath and iridologist. Allen has worked in natural medicine for almost thirty years and is known as the 'grandmother' of the industry in Western Australia. She managed to speedily source homeopathic versions of the three immune-boosting supplements mum was recommended (mistletoe, one of the substances, is difficult to get hold of in Australia).

The other natural treatment suggested for mum, Haelan, was already working a treat, according to Allen's analysis: 'I've never seen someone bounce back so well from such a serious cancer as you have,' she said, before adding: 'Maybe you should give yourself a break from tests for a bit now.' Mum quite agreed.

•

CHAPTER 11

Energy Medicine

*'Some of their rules can be bent,
others can be broken.'*
Morpheus, *The Matrix*

I f you're ever in the mood to be awe-struck, I suggest you watch
a video of a tumour being dissolved in a matter of minutes. The
healing of a three-inch diameter bladder cancer, in a woman who
has been diagnosed as inoperable, is not something you see every
day. The now famous video, which you can watch on YouTube,
illustrates the power of the mind to influence the physical body.[1]
Luke Chan recorded the phenomenal feat at a 'medicine-less'
hospital in Beijing, China, where patients are treated and cured
exclusively with chi – life energy. 'I was stunned when I video-
taped the ultrasound image of a cancerous tumour as it was
being 'removed' naturally, under the supervision of doctors,'
writes Chan in his book, *101 Miracles of Natural Healing*. 'I immediately felt that the self-healing art of Chi-Lel [a form of qigong]
must be a new frontier in fighting disease which everyone should
know about.'

Energy medicine is variously described as the 'secret of life',[2]
the 'missing piece of the healing puzzle'[3] and a 'breakthrough in
human body biological engineering'.[4] Physicist Dr Claude
Swanson, educated at MIT and Princeton University, is at the

forefront of this emerging field. Describing the latest discoveries in energy medicine, he says: 'It is called chi, prana, mana, orendo, waken, Baraka, and life force. It is the energy which enables adepts, yogis and shamen to achieve the miraculous feats they do. It enables qigong masters from China to project their energy over thousands of miles to heal injured cells and to cure cancer in laboratory experiments.'[5]

In 2007, leading qigong master Jixing Li conducted a distance-healing experiment with Pennsylvania State University Medical School. As part of the study, human leukaemia cells were grown in four flasks and arranged in incubators. Master Li, who resides in California, was asked to send healing energy to one of the flasks, labelled 'IC'. The result? At the end of the month-long experiment, no leukaemia cells were alive in IC while the control flasks – those not sent healing energy – still had an average of more than 140 million leukaemia cells alive.[6] And this is not a one-off phenomenon: British healer Matthew Manning has also proved it's possible to influence cancer cells in laboratory conditions. In one series of experiments twenty-seven out of thirty test flasks revealed drops in the cancer cell count. None of the control flasks showed any significant changes.[7]

Based on communicating with the earth's 'universal energy', Master Li's technique has proven remarkably effective at treating a wide variety of illnesses deemed impossible to cure. 'Many patients with late-stage cancer have shown marked improvement,' says Li. Yet despite decades of medical 'miracles' and mind-bending experiments, Li's work has been largely ignored by the mainstream medical community: 'Qigong experiments are often beyond the range of scientific comprehension, so they are simply ignored or written off as useless,' he explains.

But the tide is turning. Thanks to the rapid evolution in technology, we now have the tools to measure the 'subtle energies' which ancient cultures have used for centuries to heal. Dr Swanson, author of the groundbreaking *Life Force, the Scientific*

Basis, says: 'The Koreans have been able to photograph the acupuncture channels ... and they really do carry this special energy ... the life-force energy through the body,' says Swanson, adding that this measurable 'chi' energy shows us that the mind is much more powerful than we might ever have imagined.[8]

So What is Energy?

'Energy animates every cell and organ in your body,' explains Donna Eden, one of the world's best-known energy healers and author of *The Little Book of Energy Medicine.* 'It is the Life Force and, put simply: when you have it, you are alive; when you don't, you aren't.' Every breath you take, every thought you create and even the surfaces you touch have the power to alter your energy. 'The cells of living tissue are electrical direct current (DC) systems. All life generates an electrical DC charge,' explains Dr Garry Gordon, co-founder of the American College for Advancement in Medicine (ACAM).

But just as batteries wear out, so does the human energy system if it's not recharged. 'If you've got a health problem, you've got an energy problem,' says Dr Alex Loyd, creator of the Healing Codes, a technique which identifies the core emotional/energy issues that control every aspect of our lives. And for Dr Gordon, a lack of energy is a leading cause of cancer: 'It's as if you own a flashlight and the batteries are 90 per cent dead,' he says. Others agree: 'Cancer cells are universally disturbed in their electronic energy balance, an understanding that potentially revolutionises cancer therapy and prevention,' says renowned geneticist Dr Mae-Wan Ho.[9]

So what leads to disturbances in energy? Mineral deficiencies, negative attitudes, emotional trauma, electro-smog and ineffective breathing are just some ways we lose energy, according to experts. 'Negative attitudes about life diminish the life force itself.

The life force gradually, but continually, becomes weakened. The body, the mind and the spirit begin to suffer from "energy malnutrition",' writes Caroline Myss in *The Creation of Health*.

A lack of magnesium can also spell disaster for your cells. 'If you don't have magnesium you can't create energy,' says Kathryn Alexander, a naturopath based in Queensland. 'So very often if you give people magnesium they will notice improvement in their energy.'[10] And as for electronic pollution: 'Each molecule in the body has a unique shape, a unique frequency, what we call an electromagnetic radiation or EMR,' explains Dr Zenon Gruba, a conventionally trained physician from Melbourne. 'If we know that, then we can also understand why telecommunication towers are dangerous, because they're giving off distinct EMRs that are foreign to our internal communication.'

For those who slept through high-school science, energy medicine can sometimes seem impenetrable. Terms like 'mitochondrial health', 'quantum mechanics' and 'string theory' can deter those who want fast answers to serious health concerns. On the other hand, those allergic to the spiritual realm might snigger at talk of chakras, prayer and pranayama. But regardless of the language used, there's one key message that radiates: everything is energy.

In this chapter we dive right into the ever-expanding sea of energy medicine. From pulsed electromagnetic field therapy, to acupuncture and magnetic healing, I hope there is something in here that resonates with you. For mum, understanding the importance of energy – and connecting with spirit – has transformed her approach to getting well. There is a smorgasbord of energy healing tools and techniques available to the intrepid explorer, but you needn't practise them all to start improving your cellular health. Whether you decide to detach from a negative morphic field, listen to a healing frequency or start your day with an energy clearing exercise, you will be doing something to recharge your life force.

The Most Popular Form of Energy Medicine

Acupuncture can be traced back at least 3000 years to the Shang Dynasty in China, while Marco Polo reportedly brought the ancient art to the West in the 1300s.

For those who haven't tried it, this traditional Chinese medicine technique involves inserting a series of very thin needles along the energy meridians of the body to stimulate the flow of chi and restore balance. Following decades of research – including hundreds of research papers published in prestigious Western journals – we now know that acupuncture is effective at treating a host of conditions including addiction, depression, erectile dysfunction, headaches and infertility. Dr Norm Shealy, neurosurgeon and author of *Energy Medicine – the Future of Health,* has used acupuncture since 1967: 'I have found that most of the time when a woman is having a delayed period, I can start the period in less than twenty-four hours by stimulating a circuit called the Chang-Mo.' Shealy created the first doctoral programme in energy medicine and is currently Professor of the subject at Holos University.

With regards to cancer, the World Health Organisation states that acupuncture is useful for relieving pain and controlling the adverse effects of radiotherapy and chemotherapy.[11] Mum has found acupuncture to be a great way to diffuse stress; she has been seeing Dr Jerzy Dycynski, a qualified European cardiologist based in Perth, Western Australia, sporadically since her diagnosis. Dr Dycynski, or 'George' as he prefers to be called, believes that lowering stress can help uncover the protective genes that are vital to defend us from cancer. Using Cardio Stress Imaging Technology, George is able to measure the stress levels of his patients on arrival, and retest them following treatment. Recently he published a paper showing that just one acupuncture intervention was able to lower stress levels effectively in 94.6 per cent of patients.[12] For mum, simply taking the time to visit George meant paying more attention to her stress levels: 'Often I'd go to the appointment thinking I was fairly relaxed, but then George's machine would tell me otherwise,' she says.

The unconscious is more than a million times more powerful than the conscious, according to Bruce Lipton. We might *think* we're on top of things – emotionally, physically, energetically – but our bodies often tell a different story.

Grief in Your Lungs, Terror in Your Kidneys?

Paul Lennard, an energy healer based in Harley Street, London, can sense people's energy fields and can often 'see' events in a person's life that have led to physical and emotional problems. While working at a health spa in Europe, Lennard met a woman who had a severe eating disorder and was allergic to almost every type of food. 'Within two minutes of meeting her I said, "Okay, I am getting a picture of a model train set for some reason," and she replied, "Oh, that was in my lounge; that's what I used to focus on when my cousin was molesting me,"' says Lennard. 'She hadn't been able to talk about that with anyone before.' One year later, the woman sent Lennard a letter saying she was feeling so much better and had just had her first baby.[13]

When mum saw Paul Lennard during a visit to London, he asked whether she had been in a horrible car accident when she was thirteen. 'No,' mum replied. 'But I think I know what you're talking about.' When she was thirteen, two young brothers and a girl mum knew were killed in a head-on collision. Mum remembers going to the funeral and seeing the three coffins lined up together: 'It's given me a phobia of funerals ever since,' she says. But how might such a memory have been affecting mum's health? 'The memory might be stored as fear in the bladder or terror in a different organ,' says Lennard. 'So you get an emotional weakness in a certain area and then a problem comes along.'

So what does an energy session look like? I decided to book an appointment with Lennard to find out. After asking a few basic questions, I was instructed to lie down, fully clothed, on the massage table as Lennard scanned his hands over my body. I quickly began to feel a whoosh of energy circulate through my torso as memories swirled around my mind (some people go to sleep). If Lennard senses a significant 'event' in your past that needs clearing, he might ask you about it; otherwise he might approach emotional traumas through a more three-dimensional route. Using a type of deep-tissue massage called Chi Nei Tsang Lennard is able to release emotional blockages from the body. At one point I was asked to lie on my back as he zeroed in on a knot underneath my right shoulder blade. The pain was excruciating, albeit momentary. Afterwards, I realised how much easier it was to breathe; it was as if I'd been holding my breath for years. 'That would have been some kind of grief held in your lungs,' says Lennard. 'So physically I could release it rather than going into it emotionally.'

The term 'emotional baggage' may be more than a metaphorical image. When we don't fully understand or process a negative emotional experience it can, quite literally, get trapped in our bodies. 'Much of our suffering is due to negative emotional energies that have become trapped within us,' writes Dr Bradley Nelson, in his best-selling book *The Emotion Code*. Casey Terry,[14] a psychologist and reiki master based in Australia, uses various energetic tools to uncover these blockages. So how important is it to let go of our baggage? 'It can save someone's life,' says Terry. 'That blocked energy has to go somewhere, so it might form like a tumour or growth, or it might manifest as some sort of chronic emotional issue. When people start clearing this stuff they start feeling more alive and more inspired,' says Terry. Interestingly, energy healing was among the most frequently discussed treatments in the 'unexpected remission' interviews conducted by Dr Kelly Turner (see Chapter 12).

Protecting Your Energy

Returning from an energy healer can leave you feeling light, enlivened and ready to make life changes. And then reality hits. You get stuck in traffic, you read a depressing headline or you spend an hour on the phone to an energy vampire.

For mum, a simple mantra – 'It's not me, it's not mine, I surrender it to the universe' – helps to deflect negative vibes. Another phrase that helps her detach is 'infinite love and gratitude', coined by holistic healer Dr Darren Weissman. You can deploy these phrases whenever you see fit: cross paths with your ex? 'Infinite love and gratitude'; your boss's bad mood? 'It's not me, it's not mine'; your mother-in-law's subtle put-down? As spiritual technician Reverend Dr Iyanla Vanzant counsels: indulge in that bad thought – then cancel it. 'As soon as I have it, you know what I say? "Cancel, cancel." But I give myself permission to have the thought, otherwise I'm denying my own self-expression,' she says.[15] Dr Vanzant is the author of five *New York Times* bestsellers.

If your inbox is weighed down by negative energy (in the form of spam) you could try imagining nets of light around your router, while repeating the following phrase: 'I ask that platinum nets be placed on my phones and internet to deflect all negativity back to its original source. Thank you it is done, it is done, it is done!' suggests Rebecca Yates, an energy healer from Perth, who, incidentally, looks a solid ten years younger than she is (this seems to be a trend among energy healers).

In shamanic culture, it's understood that harbouring 'negative entities' or 'negative attachments' can lead to illness. To banish these invisible parasites, Tony Norgrove,[16] a shamanic healer from Western Australia, suggests visualising a purple flame for five minutes every morning. 'An attachment, shamanically speaking, is a non-belonging energy inside someone that feeds off negative energy,' he explains, adding that it doesn't take a life-threatening situation to become 'a banquet' for these attachments. 'We have 40,000 thoughts every day,' says Norgrove. 'And most of these are crap thoughts: we're worrying about the future or just worrying about what's for dinner. The more negative a person is – the more likely they are to attract these things.' Mum's neck pain literally vanished after her session with Norgrove. Mind over matter? Maybe. But imagining a 'purple flame' is certainly a lot cheaper than physio.

Refrigerating Your Foes?

Doreen Virtue, author of *How To Hear Your Angels*, has a unique suggestion for releasing any pent-up negativity and 'psychic debris'. She recommends writing down the names of people who've stung you with verbal abuse, putting the piece of paper in a plastic container of water and placing it in the freezer compartment of your refrigerator: 'You'll have an immediate sense of release as you put these names in the freezer; keep them there for a minimum of three months,' she advises. Mum loved this idea and immediately thought of all the people she would like to leave next to the ice tray. But then she exclaimed, 'Oh my God, but what if people put *me* in the freezer!' before erupting in peals of laughter.

By embracing a bit of 'woo-woo' – be it through talking to your spirit guides (as mum and I do daily), imagining a purple flame or listening to a healing frequency – you are inviting an element of playfulness into your life that is, if nothing else, fun.

The Software of Your Soul

Imagine if you could simply flick a switch in your subconscious and change your physical reality? Brent Phillips certainly thinks it's possible. 'All of us on the inside are full of software, just like a computer,' says Phillips, who graduated at the top of his class at the Massachusetts Institute of Technology. It was 'at the time of the internet boom', he says. 'I figured I would move to California, start an internet company, work really hard for a couple of years then sell the company, make millions of dollars and move to a tropical island to go hot tub with supermodels.' But it didn't work out like that. After a few years of hundred-hour working weeks, Phillips was left semi-crippled, with a frozen arm. Over the course of several years he tried everything conventional and alternative medicine had to offer, including surgery, reiki and physiotherapy – to no avail.

Desperate to find something that would improve his condition, and willing to try 'anything', Phillips eventually agreed to have a Theta Healing session, with a healer named Terry O'Connell.[17] 'The session was interesting, if nothing else. We talked about what had happened with my career ... my relationship with women and we talked about my relationship with God. But the whole time, I was kind of going "What does this have to do with my arm?" At the end of the session Terry[18] was like, "Okay Brent. We're going to do a healing now." She kind of closed her eyes and went into a trance. After a minute or two I actually felt something, like, popped in my elbow. It was the weirdest thing and she opened her eyes and said, "Try your arm".'

Needless to say, Phillips found he was able to move his arm, previously declared 'permanent and stationary' by doctors. That was the start of his new career as a Theta Healer. Over the last few years Phillips has helped hundreds of clients overcome everything from allergies and asthma to cancer and HIV ('I have had more than one client go to an undetectable viral load'). But perhaps the most remarkable healing took place on his mother. In 2010 Karen Phillips was diagnosed with clear-cell endometrial cancer. 'That's one of the really bad ones,' stresses Phillips. 'They call it a death sentence.' Before undergoing scheduled surgery, Karen Phillips had a one-hour Theta Healing session with her son over the phone. 'We cleared maybe a dozen subconscious emotional blocks she had,' Phillips says. When Karen went back and had the surgery, although there were still cancer cells found in the tissue removed, all of the clear cells – the ones that make the cancer so deadly – were gone. 'Literally all it takes to dissolve a tumour or heal a broken bone or any condition is to simply change the signal that's creating it. When you do that, it disappears,' says Phillips.

So will everyone leave a Theta Healing session sans insomnia, cancer and obesity? 'Sometimes you get miracles, sometimes you get a process,' qualifies Phillips. 'So for example, I have not yet seen anyone lose fifty or a hundred pounds overnight, but what will happen is, when you clear the subconscious blocks to being thin, you will bring into your life whatever you need to achieve that. And so for some people that might be finding a new exercise programme or a good nutritional counsellor or it might be they get a new job or move out of a toxic environment.'

The Frequency of Love

We all know music has the power to transform our state of mind, get us 'in the mood' and motivate us – a little Annie Lennox in the morning tends to set me up for the day. But did you know a single musical note can actually repair DNA? The frequency – 528 Hz – is one of the notes on the ancient Solfeggio scale, once sung in Gregorian chants and thought to impart tremendous spiritual blessings during religious masses. The scale – which mysteriously disappeared around AD 1050 – was recently re-discovered by the late Dr Joseph Puleo; 528 Hz has since been coined 'the frequency of love' and has been shown to have remarkable healing effects.

In a series of experiments, DNA was exposed to four styles of music, including Gregorian chants using the Solfeggio scale. The effects of the music were measured by looking at the DNA test-tube samples' absorption of UV light. The result? The Gregorian chants led to a marked increase in the absorption of UV light, while rock music had little or no effect.[19] Why would this be? Leading pharmacologist Dr Candace Pert sheds some light on the matter. She states that energy and vibration affect us on a molecular level. In *Molecules of Emotion* Dr Pert writes, '... we have seventy different receptors on the molecules and when vibration and frequency reach that far they begin to vibrate'. In other words our very cells begin to shimmy, when they're exposed to healing sounds.

Mum gets her daily dose of 528 Hz through Dr Alex Loyd's Master Key recording. The sound is somewhere between the hum of a phone left off the hook and the singing of a wet finger on a wine glass – but it's relaxing rather than annoying! To listen to the sacred tone, simply type 528 Hz into YouTube and you'll come across various videos with the tone.

Electronic Fields for Brain Cancer

While some believe the human body is encoded with all the necessary 'technology' to heal itself, others put their trust in man-made devices. In 2011 the US FDA approved a device for use in brain cancer which uses electrical fields to interrupt cancer cell division. In a recent TED talk, Bill Doyle, Executive Chair of Novocure (the company responsible for developing the groundbreaking therapy) discussed the benefits of the new approach.

'The [Tumour Treating Fields] patients undergo all the activities of their daily life. There's none of the tiredness. There's none of what is called the "chemo head",'[20] he says.

Melanomas have been shown to self-destruct when exposed to nanosecond pulsed electric fields. In one study published in the 2006 edition of *Biochemical and Biophysical Research Communications*, melanomas shrank by 90 per cent within two weeks.[21] For Dr Garry Gordon, electrical currents only hold part of the answer to healing. The other key component is magnetic. 'The earth's electromagnetic field has dropped from nearly 30 gauss at the time of the dinosaurs to 0.3 gauss today,' says Dr Gordon. 'These major earth changes tie into everything from chronic fatigue and depression to cancer and obesity.' How? you might well ask. 'Magnetic fields affect the nervous and circulatory systems of every living cell – animal, human and plant,' explains Dr Gordon.

Magnetic healing is nothing new – in fact, it's been around since the 1600s. Medieval healers used natural magnetic rocks called 'lodestones' to treat a variety of ailments, according to California-based physician Dr Robert Jay Rowen. However, with rapid technological advancements, magnets are back on the medical agenda. Dr Jonathan Wright started treating individuals with high-gauss magnetic field therapy in 2004 at his Tahoma Clinic in the Seattle area: 'High-gauss magnetic fields "speed up" electron flow dramatically,' says Dr Wright.

Then there is PEMF – pulsed electromagnetic field therapy – dubbed the 'revolutionary cure for pain' on the popular *Dr Oz Show*. Evidence suggests it might benefit cancer patients too: 'PEMF is going to make everything else you're doing with your exercise, your diet, your positive thinking so much better because it increases cellular oxygen levels, improves the uptake of nutrients and stimulates lymphatic flow,' says Dr Garry Gordon.

PEMF is currently the subject of intense research: there are thousands of university papers on its value, it is FDA approved[22] and even NASA has analysed its effect on stem cells. 'PEMF is one treatment everyone needs,' says Dr Rowen, adding that while previously beyond the price range of most people, it is now available cheaply with a small home unit.

Testing Your Energy

Health screening just got a whole lot more exciting. In the last few years biofeedback devices have cropped up in doctors' offices providing clients with scarily accurate information about their bodies and minds. These tools operate like a virus scan on a computer, picking up the 'energy signatures' of bacteria, parasites and mineral deficiencies eating away at your health.

During the process of writing this book I received an email from an Australian man who told me he was treating his tumour with something called a QXCI/SCIO machine. 'Interesting . . . ' I thought, then forgot all about it. Until a few weeks later, when a woman in mum's astrology class, Tamara Gries, turned up with a strange-looking contraption. Mum was blown away by the information the machine picked up and booked in for a SCIO session with Gries. After getting hooked up to the machine – by attaching wrist and ankle straps and a cyber-headband – mum watched as various areas of her body lit up the screen.

'If something comes up, it means there's an energy disturbance in that area,' says Gries, a Perth-based holistic practitioner. Mum's adrenal glands, crown chakra and lymph system flashed repeatedly. 'No surprises there,' mum said. 'I had thirteen lymph nodes taken out when I had the hysterectomy.' What was surprising though was the measles vaccine 'tag' that appeared: a vaccination

▶

mum had been given over twenty years ago. So what does the patient do with all this information? 'The SCIO sends a biofeedback frequency to stabilise those areas in your body,' Gries explained.

For the diagnosis of chronic disease sophisticated blood analyses (see Chapter 10) cannot be matched. But for a snapshot of a patient's general well-being, biofeedback might be more illuminating. 'I used to routinely perform blood tests and then I was introduced to the biofeedback,' says Dr Diane Meyer, dentist, psychologist and author of *Pick Your Poisons*. 'After that, I was doing both the blood tests and the biofeedback to identify nutritional deficiencies – and getting the same results. Now I have turned a little bit away from the blood . . . and I leave it up to the individual to choose whatever resonates with them.' For the needle phobic that's brilliant news; it's also the perfect option for those, like mum and I, who love a bit of navel gazing.

Mother Nature's Energy

The ground is alive with powerful healing electrons which help balance our body and keep us healthy: 'It's thought that the influx of free electrons from the Earth's surface will help to neutralise free radicals and reduce both acute and chronic inflammation, which is at the root of many health conditions and accelerated ageing,' explains legendary natural health expert Dr Joseph Mercola, in a recent article.

For Marcus Freudenmann, producer of *CANCER is Curable NOW*, walking barefoot on the grass or the beach not only offsets free radical damage but also stops red blood cells from clotting.

Mum was the first to alert me to the importance of connecting with the earth: 'The American Indians believe that when we began building footpaths, roads and driving everywhere in cars, we lost not only our connection with the earth but we lost our ability to heal ourselves,' she says.

Rather than regularly plugging into the ground, today we constantly connect with wireless devices, cordless phones and computers, which have the potential to wreak havoc on our health. Is 'earthing' the answer? Studies in peer-reviewed journals suggest that it just might be. One report found that ' ... when the human body is grounded it is naturally protected from static electricity and radiated electric fields'.[23] Further evidence suggests that earthing can reduce muscle pain, provide antioxidant protection, balance the hormonal system oxygenate the blood.[24]

But even if you don't kick off your shoes, just getting outside is good for you. We intuitively know that walking beneath a canopy of branches, listening to the rustle of leaves and breathing in fresh air quenches the soul. Sadly, many of us are natur-exics. A British survey conducted in 2010 by the Royal Society for the Protection of Birds[25] found that only 37 per cent of under thirty-fives feel connected to the natural world. Despite this, 76 per cent of respondents said that being out in nature was a great stress reducer and more than half said they need time in nature to be happy. Kids instinctively recognise the need for nature. A report by Natural England revealed that 81 per cent of children would love more outside play.

Heal the Earth, Heal Yourself?

More than a breath of fresh air, the natural environment is literally our lungs, our energry source – without trees there would be no oxygen; without healthy soil almost one third of all living organisms[26] would disappear; it's the start – and end – of our food chain. The earth is literally our energy source; it's the start – and end – of our food chain. We easily forget this fact as we go about our busy important lives, hunched over screens in incubated offices. But if we want to stay healthy, we can't afford to stay inside, according to Master Li. He believes that connecting with and giving back to Mother Nature is *the* key to healing.

When he's not proving the 'impossible' – telepathically transferring images, influencing the weather or healing chronic illness – Master Li is planting trees. The main aim of his 'Universal Energy Foundation' is to improve and protect the ecosystem. He suggests on his website that donating to his foundation will improve your health. How, you might well ask? I spoke to Master Li's student, Joan, to find out: 'When someone is ill it's usually because they are not living in balance and harmony with nature – it could be that they're still on their computer at twelve at night when they should be asleep or it could be that they are not connecting and giving back to the Mother Earth,' she explains. To help bring the person back in balance, Master Li always donates some of the patient's fee to his environmental foundation. And this is not simply a ploy to further his own philanthropy – Master Li has been known to waive a patient's fee, as long as they promise to donate to *some* environmental organisation to help themselves heal.

I've been moved to see the connection between healing ourselves and healing the planet many times in the process of writing this book. Two renowned writers and cancer survivors, Marc Ian Barasch and Professor Jane Plant both invested more energy in the environment after recovering from cancer. In 2005 Barasch, a prolific author, magazine editor and producer, founded the Green World Campaign which aims to turn degraded lands green again. For her part, Professor Plant writes at the end of her book *Your Life in Your Hands* ' . . . I am increasingly concerned with the environment and the sustainability of the surface of the beautiful blue planet called Earth as a place to live. Breast cancer changed me ... It made me stop. And smell the (wild) roses.'

To stay healthy, Master Li encourages everyone to invite nature's healing energies into the body, on a daily basis. 'The morning is the best time of day, the energy is best,' says Joan. 'Just sit there, in a place filled with trees and welcome it. You don't need to put out any requests or intentions – just open yourself and send your appreciation to Mother Nature.'

Feeling 'appreciation' in the body has now been shown in laboratory experiments to alter our chemical composition. 'When we are able to hold, what to us is appreciation or gratitude ... our brain signals our body to release the life-affirming chemicals,' writes Gregg Braden in *The Isaiah Effect*. 'What our own science is able to digitally measure and acknowledge is that we create coherence in our body through the quality of feeling we hold in our heart.'

Feeling-based Prayer

This is quite a radical departure from the way many of us think of prayer. I previously associated the ritual with pleading, desperation and negotiation: a mother on her knees imploring God to save her sick child or a promise to be better if only the bleak situation changed. But if you believe Gregg Braden, this is not the most effective way to pray. If there's something you want to achieve, whether it's vibrant health or a better relationship, the key is to *feel* as though it's already happened. 'The technology of prayer stems from our ability to choose which thoughts, feelings and emotions we embody in the moment,' explains Braden. You might choose to recall the last time you had a deep belly laugh with a friend and infuse a current fear with that immediate sense of joy, or perhaps fill your body with stillness and peace simply by remembering the theme tune to a cherished childhood sit-com.

Many cancer patients and their families turn to prayer following a diagnosis, and while sceptics continue to trash the concept of prayer and healing, it seems heaven is louder. A *Time*/CNN poll[27] discovered that 82 per cent of Americans believe that prayer can cure serious illness, 73 per cent believe that prayer for others works – and 64 per cent want their physicians to pray for them. And doctors aren't afraid to ask for God's helping hand: 99 per cent of physicians are convinced that religious beliefs can heal, according to a *Lancet* report.

Once, when mum arrived at Dr 'George's' office in a particularly anxious frame of mind, he asked her: 'Can we pray together for you?' Dr George knelt beside the bed where mum was lying, covered in acupuncture needles, and said something to the effect of: 'We ask the Lord to help Gemma find healing and release the stress from her body.' This isn't the first time someone has offered to pray for mum. A few weeks into starting the blog I received this message from David, a distance healer living in LA: 'Without your mum's permission I would not act, but I would like to ... add her name to our distant-healing register and request that our group of 50+ healers send her healing.'

Referring to distance healing, Dr Keith Scott-Mumby, author of *Cancer Research Secrets*, states: 'In contrast to relying on a word phrase, experienced healers usually focus upon a feeling state of love and connect to the heart of the target person.' This idea that prayer is a feeling is echoed by countless others. 'Most of us will say prayer is just about putting your hands together and appealing to something greater than yourself. But there's a deeper point to it,' says Bryan Hubbard, co-publisher of the health journal *What Doctors Don't Tell You*. 'I think fundamentally prayer is trying to demonstrate that somehow there is this unity. When you feel that sense of unity and love, the body's immune system kick-starts back into life.'

Hubbard recently wrote a special report on prayer. It revealed that prayer, reiki and other distant-healing therapies do appear to work, even if researchers are at a loss to understand why. In a review of 350 prayer studies (double-blinded, peer-reviewed and randomised) researchers found that 75 per cent demonstrated that prayer had a positive impact, 17 per cent found it had no impact and 7 per cent showed a negative impact.

But arguing over whether prayer really works might be missing the point. Ultimately, if it feels good – do it. 'When I get up in the morning, my prayer is, "Dear God, let me make someone in your universe laugh today",' says Dr Zenon Gruba. 'I reckon if we can all do that, we'd be like ripples on a pond, we'd resonate with one another, those ripples would get bigger and stronger and then we'd have the perfect tsunami of feel-good energy.' Although there is no prescription for prayer, it's worth remembering this key point: whether you're reciting the Lord's prayer, performing salat or chanting a Hindu mantra, what falls from your lips might be less important than what you feel in your body.

Mum fully believes that divine intervention has helped her heal: 'When I was diagnosed with cancer I connected with spirit in a big way,' she says. 'Having grown up Catholic, prayer came easily to me, but I also called upon spirit guides, archangels and asked them for help all the time. And believe it or not, I received it.' Mum converses daily with her spirit guide 'Serene' and regularly calls on archangels Michael and Raphael for healing (and occasionally Jophiel, the archangel of beauty, if she wants her hair to look good). But mum also acknowledges that our earthly actions are vital. 'You've got to co-create,' she quipped the other day. In other words, there's no point praying if you're going to procrastinate. You also need to nourish your body with the right foods, ensure you're getting enough oxygen, pull out the poisons and take whatever medicines or treatments resonate with you.

May the Force Be With You

Some believe that in viewing the body as a machine with separate, malfunctioning parts, modern medicine is fundamentally flawed. I tend to agree. But that's not to say that if I broke my l eg, developed bacterial meningitis or was in a car accident that I wouldn't be desperate to get to the hospital as soon as Newtonian speed allowed. Sometimes even a headache will only respond to paracetamol. Allopathic medicine will always have a place, but it doesn't have all the answers.

For Dr Norm Shealy the role of energy medicine is clear: 'When there is no need for surgery or a life-saving drug, and especially when the condition becomes chronic or when the medical therapy recommended is extremely toxic and poses great risks, I think patients have a responsibility to evaluate and decide about the potential of energy medicine to provide comfort and healing.'

Energy medicine is a vast universe of divine sound, light frequencies and overlapping realities; it's where space-age machinery and shamanic healing exist in tandem and imagination holds court. In this chapter I have only scratched the surface. There are many other energy techniques including tapping, kinesiology and the Journey process that are equally deserving of attention. But then it's not my intention to provide an exhaustive account; rather, I hope to have piqued your interest and given you some practical ways to fuel your cells and light up your spirit.

CHAPTER 12

●

Inspiring Stories

*'Tell me a fact and I'll listen, tell me a truth
and I'll hear, but tell me a story
and it will live in my heart forever.'*
Native American Indian wisdom

It started with an email: 'I also said no to chemo' read the subject line. I eagerly opened it and devoured the story.

So often we hear from cancer survivors who have chosen the conventional route; newspapers and magazines are filled with testimonials from patients who've endured the rigours of conventional treatment and come out the other side. However, those who have taken the natural path are rarely given a voice. People are – rightfully – scared of putting cure and 'not having chemo' in the same sentence. So instead of being quizzed about their experience, natural cancer survivors are often hushed up and dismissed, their hard-earned recovery muddied by accusations of 'misdiagnosis' and their return to health heralded as a 'miracle' – an equally diminishing and unhelpful word which denies their active role in getting well.

In the academic literature, a cancer recovery that occurs in the absence of allopathic medicine is referred to as a 'spontaneous remission'. Researchers have estimated that spontaneous remission (SR) occurs in one out of every 60,000 to 100,000 cancer patients. However, this estimate fails to take into account those individuals who decided not to return to their conventional doctor after getting well. It also overlooks under-reporting. Not all physicians take the time to write and submit potential cases of spontaneous remission, particularly if they are at a loss to understand why it occurred.

With a dearth of research on the subject, New York-based cancer counsellor and researcher Dr Kelly Turner decided to make it the subject of her doctoral thesis. What she discovered was so fascinating her work is now being turned into a book entitled *Unexpected Remission*. 'An unexpected remission is a cancer remission that occurs either without conventional medical treatment, after conventional treatment has failed to work or when conventional and complementary methods are used in conjunction to overcome a dire prognosis,' Dr Turner explains. Her thesis might have riled the medical community, but it's catnip for the cancer traveller. 'I'm glad it's reaching cancer patients and friends and family of cancer patients, because that's whom I wrote it for,' says Dr Turner. Her research led her on a global quest, in the course of which she met Japanese oncologists who believe bacteria are to blame and African practitioners who receive guidance in their dreams. After interviewing twenty subjects who defied a death sentence and talking to over fifty physicians and healers, Dr Turner found common threads lined the path to recovery. The six most frequently mentioned treatments or beliefs were as follows:

1 Deepening one's spirituality

2 Trusting in intuition regarding health decisions

3 Releasing suppressed emotions

4 Feeling love/joy/happiness

5 Changing one's diet

6 Taking herbal or vitamin supplements

Commenting on the results, Dr Turner says: 'We've all heard about faith healings and so I was certainly ready for this topic [spirituality] to come up,' she says. 'But what I wasn't expecting is that ... people weren't describing a spiritual belief, but rather a spiritual experience or energy.' Instead of simply 'believing in Jesus', Turner's subjects spoke of finding a deep inner peace. 'What my findings imply is that you have to find a spiritual or even a *relaxation* practice that brings a change about in your body,' she says.

We now know, beyond a shadow of doubt, that our thoughts and feelings affect our biochemistry. When we're feeling anxious, for example, we secrete the stress hormone adrenaline, which has been shown in studies to make cancer resistant to treatment. But by choosing to stop fear-driven thoughts and finding a healing space in our minds we can take control. 'If you look at all the studies on experienced meditators, what we find is that when they reach deep levels of meditation, their entire physiology changes,'[1] says Turner. 'As soon as they start really deeply connecting in that meditative state, their glands start secreting serotonin, dopamine, oxytocin ... all of these wonderful things, which we know from other studies, really help the immune system.' For some of Kelly's subjects 'deepening one's spirituality' meant waking up with the sunrise, for others it meant whirling around like the famous 'whirling dervishes' – but whatever the chosen practice, it caused subjects to feel a shift in their bodies.

While the importance of spirituality may not have come as a surprise to Dr Turner, 'Trusting in intuition' did: 'Wasn't that interesting?' she says. 'Whenever I give lectures and I get to that slide, I say: "I have to tell you, I was not expecting this one to come up – I was really expecting exercise",' says Turner, hastening to add that while exercise wasn't a priority when the subjects first embarked on their healing journey, as their strength grew, it became more important.

In the current climate, following gut feelings about health might seem radical, even reckless. But following doctors' orders doesn't always work either: 'A lot of my subjects had tried chemo and radiation and their immune systems were so ravaged ... they needed deeper, quieter things that led them to their healing and intuition was one of them,' Dr Turner explains. For some people that meant following their instincts with regard to herbal supplements and therapies, but for others it meant changing something in their life that was hampering their recovery: 'I have some people who swear up and down that their diet change alone did it. I have other people who changed their diet the same way – nothing happened; but lo and behold they left their emotionally abusive relationship and they got well,' says Turner.

The word 'intuition' came up a lot in my own survivor interviews, and for mum, trusting her instincts has also been vital: 'I have tried many things and many approaches, some of which I have discarded along the way,' she says. 'Many experts believed for me to get on top of my cancer I must give up meat, become vegan. Intuitively, this just didn't feel right for me, so I didn't do it. Instead, I try to choose meat that is grass-fed, organic, antibiotic and hormone-free. However, when I was told to give up dairy, regrettably this did feel right, and I have not looked back.'

Rarely, however, do people rely on intuition alone. You need only look at the Amazon history on mum's computer to know that a huge amount of research helped pave her recovery. Others have said the same: 'The reason that I personally did not go down the chemo route was not just an instinctive reaction,' says Vincent Crewe who reversed advanced colon cancer. 'I had done much research into chemotherapy and what I learned convinced me it was not the route for me to take.' Jessica Richards, natural breast cancer survivor and author of *The Topic of Cancer*, also shared with me her decision process: 'I would like to make it very clear that I did not base any of my choices on belief. I simply made rational decisions based on the facts and evidence presented to me in that I did everything I could to support my immune system (rather than destroy it) and at the same time, wreck the cancer environment within my body.' Jessica was recommended a partial or full mastectomy and removal of lymph nodes, intensive chemo, radiotherapy and five years of drugs. Instead, she chose to change her diet and mental attitude and had various treatments including intravenous vitamin C.

Since I started the blog, various readers have contacted me to share the importance of working with, rather than against their cancer: 'Partnering with your body is the way to healing. I am big on supporting cells so that they can thrive,' says Sandra Hornsby-White, long-term natural cancer survivor and holistic health-care practitioner. Lee Gefen, who was diagnosed with a rare brain tumour at thirty-two, has similar thoughts: 'I no longer feel like the tumour is threatening me, or invading me or that I have to fight it. I am learning to live with it in peace, while doing everything I can to treat what caused it in the first place.'

This stands in sharp contrast to the conventional approach, which often uses warlike metaphors: 'Doctors talk about hitting the tumour hard, of going in aggressively. We talk of people battling cancer and of losing their battle with cancer. Sadly, too many patients become the victims of that war, not the victors,' says mum, who has worked very hard not to see her cancer as the enemy. Dr Turner found this a common theme among her subjects: 'So many of the people I interviewed who have had these amazing healings – they don't talk about killing their cancer – they talk about healing their cells and healing their immune systems,' she says. One of her research interviewees, a Japanese man who overcame stage-4 cancer, sent love to his cancer every day. 'He said that he imagined his cancer was a child – his child – whom he had neglected via his work, stress and lack of sleep and who now needed his love and attention,' says Dr Turner. The man healed himself naturally after chemotherapy and surgery did not work; he changed his personal belief system, began humming, singing and chanting and let go of his fear of death. Twenty-four years later, he is still cancer-free.

When Dr Turner asked people why they healed, the answers were illuminating. 'A belief that surprised me was the idea that you have to change the underlying conditions and then cancer just simply won't be able to grow,' says Turner. 'It became the reason for changing your diet, the reason for changing your mental state.'

Recurrence is the number-one fear for anyone who's reached remission. However, Dr Turner found that by targeting the root cause, her subjects were less afraid of the cancer coming back. 'In traditional cancer treatment, you get your treatment and then ... you're sort of waiting for that five-year mark, whereas the people I met were saying: "I've turned my cancer around by doing this, this, and this – I've changed the milieu of my body, so cancer simply can't grow any more, so I'm no longer worried about recurrence."'

Change seems to be the 'open sesame' for recovery, whether you embrace conventional medicine or choose the alternative path. When researchers from MD Anderson in Texas looked at survivors who had experienced unexplained survival time after being told their condition was terminal, they found a willingness to take action was key.[2] One participant said of their illness: 'It really made me wake up and ... put a different perspective on life where I appreciate things more.'

Seeing cancer as a wake-up call is undoubtedly more life-affirming than seeing yourself as a prisoner of the condition: 'A lot of cancer patients I meet who aren't doing so well feel that everything is a punishment and that everything they have to do – from juicing kale to having chemo – is something they don't want,' says Turner. 'A lot of them are resisting change; they just want to go back to their old life.'

A willingness to discard old diets, habits and thought patterns, was common among the survivors I spoke to, even as the practical steps on their journeys diverged. In this chapter you will hear from a young Australian woman who cured herself of breast cancer using a black salve and raw-food diet, a German man who treated his pancreatic cancer with homeopathy, an English woman who chose apricot kernels over chemotherapy and others who, like mum, chose a smorgasbord of treatments.

The stories might be as different as night and day, but these people are no different from you. They have experienced the panic, fear and despair and chosen to focus on what they can do, rather than dwell on what they've lost. There is no recipe for success – each person must tread their own path to wellness – but rather than staring hopelessly at statistics, wouldn't it be better to read field notes from fellow travellers?

Rachel Kierath, Australia: diagnosed 2011, aged 31 – stage-3 breast cancer

Once I got past the fear . . . I knew I could beat it, and do it my way.

'My partner and I were waiting to see a movie, when he just sort of said, "I don't know how to bring this up, but I actually think you need to get a breast check," implying that he'd found a lump.

'When I went to have the ultrasound, I wasn't overly concerned. I had previously been told I was too young to warrant having check-ups. However, it became immediately apparent that something was wrong. "Look, we want to do a biopsy," the nurse told me, after a team of concerned staff came into the room. I was just thinking, No, this can't be. This is not right.

'The following Monday my GP called me in. I was an absolute wreck; I just knew, so sitting there listening to my doctor deliver the news that I knew he was going to deliver, was such a torment. I mean, it was only two years since my mum had passed away from breast cancer, and I had my two kids out in the waiting room, so the way it happened . . . was just this horrible mess.

'I guess the unfortunate thing was I'd just had enough of cancer, you know? Mum spent sixteen years fighting her battle. So there I am, thirty-one years of age, having just recently gone through a divorce and having lost mum. It was a time when I'd had to regroup and reassess life. I was just feeling like I'd gotten everything the way I wanted, I'd bounced back and it was time for me again, I had a new relationship . . . only to feel like it was all being taken away from me.

'I ended up seeing the same medical team that my mum had because they were considered the best. So that was a bit difficult – going to all these appointments with my dad at the same hospital, with the same people that we'd seen with mum. When I went to see the surgeon, she pretty much gave it to me straight. She told me that with a cancer of this nature, with it being so aggressive, and my age, the prognosis was likely very poor and that she would recommend chemo, essentially as a life extension.

'All the doctors were saying to me it's the "only way to go". Even my family was uncomfortable about me declining chemo, even after all we had witnessed with mum. But in the end, I had to say to myself: "Stop! You know there are so many other options out there, you *know* it doesn't work," and I just had to edit out what I was hearing, just go back to what I knew and had researched. I ended up digging out all of mum's files, my files of research I'd packed away, reminding myself of what I knew to be true and all the therapies and supplements that had started to work for mum.

'The very first thing that I did was switch to a completely raw diet. Food literally became medicine. It was not anything to be consumed because of enjoyment; it was purely a medicine. I also started taking a whole bunch of herbs known to have strong anti-cancer properties and I started taking a concoction called cansema [the internal version of black salve; see Livia's story, page 247].

'I started this regime ten days before I was due to go in for surgery. In that time, all my tumours had, on average, halved. Amazing, right? The surgeons downplayed it though; their reaction was, "Oh well, you know, ultrasound measurements aren't always that accurate." But we're talking about ultrasound measurements that can measure a foetus and tell you exactly when your due date is. Now don't tell me they're not accurate!

'With the new pathology results, all of a sudden my outlook, my prognosis, went from being really poor to being told I have this really good fighting chance of beating it. But I still had a lot of pressure to go the conventional route. If I wasn't going to have chemo, I was told to "at least do radiation". I had to sit down and explain to my oncologist, "Thanks, but no thanks." Although she was looking at me like I was a complete crazed lunatic, she knew mum's experience, so she was understanding, and what has eventuated is a nice, respectful relationship between us.

'After the surgery I bombarded my body with as much nutrition as I could. It was quite complex, but the essence of it was: I had copious amounts of vegetables – as many different colours as I could, juices, green smoothies, wheatgrass, seaweeds, all sorts of nutrient-dense foods. I limited my fruit intake, completely cut out sugar and wheat and felt an amazing transformation. I'm prone to keloid scars, but with my diet, they all regressed. I was feeling great and it was all going along just fine, and then I discovered I was pregnant.

'"There is no way you can have this baby", I was told. "You are two months out of surgery for a very aggressive breast cancer; you cannot go through with this."

'I was under an incredible amount of pressure, like you wouldn't believe, to terminate the pregnancy. I was essentially told that if I went ahead with it, I would be signing my death warrant. What I hadn't realised is that certain parts of your immune system are suppressed when you're pregnant, in order for your body not to reject the baby. So I was going to have to go into a nine-month period with a suppressed immune system, while trying to make sure that there are no stray cancer cells in my body.

'The pregnancy also meant I had to stop some of the other alternative treatments I'd started, like IV vitamin C and ozone. Even the enemas I had begun in my detoxification programme weren't recommended. I was just thinking, This is a nightmare, how am I going to do this? But the idea of terminating the pregnancy . . . it totally went against my values and I thought, How am I going to deal with the emotional fallout of terminating a child, and the consequential stress of that?

'I knew full well the link between stress and cancer and had witnessed it with mum, so I had really made an effort to reduce my own stress: I got into meditation in a big way and I gave up my position as a lecturer of Fine Arts at Curtin University, so I could focus on myself. But as I stressed about what to do with this huge dilemma, all the good work was unravelling and, three or four months into my pregnancy, the cancer came back.

'Interestingly, I found it myself. I had been for a check-up one week before where three of my medical team had given me a physical breast check and told me I was fine. But I am so in tune with my body now that I knew something was off. I just didn't feel right. I felt a dip in energy and I was also aware of a dull pain in my mastectomy site. So I spent a really good amount of time one night doing a breast check – and I found it. It was so small and so early, my surgeon commented when she actually excised it on just how unusual it was to be removing a tumour that tiny. So I'd literally found it as soon as it had started, which was lucky, because of course, with all the pregnancy hormones, the cancer would absolutely thrive, I was told.

'The recurrence confirmed to everyone that I *must* terminate the pregnancy. And, when they realised that wasn't going to happen, I was told that if I pressed ahead with the baby I would *have* to have chemo. I knew … once I got past the fear of the cancer, I knew I could beat that, and do it, my way. But with a pregnancy in the mix? That just tipped me out of my league. So I was pretty much convinced at this stage I had to have chemo, even though it went against all my instincts and research. I mean, when you're pregnant you can't have coffee, can't have alcohol, but hey, you can have chemotherapy, apparently.

'Finally, the day before I was due to start [chemo] I just thought, You know what, I've got to listen to what's true for me. When I thought about chemo, I felt utterly defeated, my energies zapped and I thought, If I don't have a lot of time left, do I really want to live my present like that? I couldn't think of anything worse than being sick all day and then trying to find the energy to fight it. I just couldn't fathom the idea. So as soon as I made the decision to go with my gut instinct – which was to reject that and do things my way – it was just this *huge* weight off my shoulders, and I knew that I had just released myself from all that stress and that I would be all right.

'But I knew there was still a lot of work to do. The recurrence made me think, Okay, clearly there's something else I'm still doing wrong – what is it? I had to go back and reassess everything that I'd been doing and also conduct some more research. Among others, I came across Professor Jane Plant's book *Your Life in Your Hands* and I really liked it because I guess, being an academic myself, I really respected and resonated with the way she tackled the subject. And of course, what she had written just made so much sense: give up dairy. Although I was on a raw diet I was still eating some yoghurt and some white cheese when the recurrence happened. Funnily enough, when I had consumed dairy before [in the early stages of pregnancy], the next morning I would inevitably be sick. But after giving up dairy? I went through the whole pregnancy feeling amazing. Normally when

I'm pregnant I'm lacking in energy and have morning sickness the whole way through, but this time it was like I wasn't even pregnant! I kept up exercise and I was jogging until I was about seven months pregnant; I had abundant energy rather than morning sickness.

'At every point in the journey, I guess the important thing has been to listen to my heart – it's always been the right choice. I put my PhD on hold, gave up my full-time job, which as a single parent was a scary decision, but it allowed me to look after myself. With both kids at school, I had between the hours of nine and three to indulge in me! I'd go outside on to the deck and get my vitamin D, listen to music or meditation CDs, prepare healthy food without being pushed for time ... I've got to say from something horrible, my everyday reality became a beautiful one. I guess it freed up the time for me to focus on all the things in life that we know we should do, but we don't.

'Of course, in lots of ways it's been hard. I've thought to myself, If I'm going to take this approach, and if I want to survive, I can't mourn my old life, because my old life led me to cancer, and if I go back to that I'm going to end up in the same position. So these changes I've made are changes for life. It's not just, Well, I'll do these things to get me through, then I'll go back to my old ways once cured, which is what my mum did, and sure enough the cancer came back.

'In so many ways it's bittersweet for me because I know that if mum hadn't had cancer and if I hadn't started looking into alternative research, there is no way I would have beaten this. It's been an amazing journey and the most important thing I'd take from it is how important it is to listen to what's true for you, rather than taking on board what's true for everyone else, whether they be doctors, whether they be family – whoever. It was almost a year to the day [from the diagnosis] that I received the all-clear. My cancer count is not only normal, it's at the *lowest* end of normal. And of course, now my two girls have what we were told was impossible: a healthy, cancer-free mother *and* a beautiful, healthy baby brother.'

Vincent Crewe, UK: diagnosed 2007, aged 57 – metastatic colon cancer

It is so important to take control and responsibility for your own health.

'As a non-drinking, non-smoking fella who had exercised most of his life, the diagnosis was a bit of a shock, to put it mildly.

'However, I have always been prone to stress, and the year before I had experienced a very tragic bereavement. My ex-wife was involved in a serious car accident – she had been hit by a guy who was speeding down a dual carriageway on the wrong side of the road. She went into a deep coma, and died a few weeks later. Telling my son Rob who was sixteen at the time that his mum wasn't coming back was the worst thing I've ever had to experience. What made it even more traumatic was that the driver got away with it. He managed to get off claiming an epileptic fit. So all that real anger, emotion that you feel – it doesn't help, does it? So it was a very difficult period and it was shortly after that that I started getting problems.

'I booked myself in for all sorts of blood tests, but there was no sign that anything was wrong. Finally, I had an examination with a camera. I distinctly remember the specialist saying, "I don't expect to find anything, but we'll have a look." What they found was a large tumour in the colon and that the cancer had spread to my liver.

'Avoiding surgery was not an option (the colon was almost completely blocked), but I knew enough about chemotherapy to want to avoid it completely. Although the oncologist tried his best to persuade me to have it, I refused flatly. When I told him

about the alternative treatments that I would be using instead –
all of which were non-toxic – he remarked arrogantly that none
of these had any proven benefits. I did point out that neither has
chemotherapy, which did not go down too well, and I could see
there was no point in discussing this with him any further and
so I took my leave. I have not been back to a hospital since that
time.

'I knew what I had to do, which was to address the toxicity,
deficiency and stress – all these elements can contribute to
cancer. But where to start? In the beginning I looked at everything that had the 'C' word attached to it: some of the stuff
resonated with me and some of it didn't and I think that's what
you've got to do; you've got to try and follow your instincts.

'Emotional toxicity is probably the hardest thing to deal with,
but I found that listening to a subliminal audio CD entitled
Powerful Immune System from a company called Inner Talk helped
with that. Every night, from the first day in the hospital, I played
it on repeat until I fell asleep and it was still playing to my subconscious as I slept.

'I also bought a book by Dr Sherry Rogers entitled *Detoxify or
Die* and that book became my bible. I learned just how toxic our
modern world is and how this can lead to serious illness. The
book also explains how to go about getting toxins out of the
body, and it was through Dr Rogers that I first learned about
coffee enemas [see Chapter 5]. Obviously you're clumsy with
everything when you start, but I soon got the hang of it and it's
the best thing I ever did.

'For the first two years I did a coffee enema every day, without
fail. There's no point putting clean petrol into a dirty tank – that
was my philosophy! Once the cancer cells started dying off, I
wanted to have all the elimination channels working as
effectively as possible. I wanted to get rid of all the residue of
anaesthetics, painkillers and morphine, lingering from the operation and I also knew that the enemas would help kick-start my

immune system too as coffee enemas can increase glutathione production.

'Now, six years on, I still do them twice a week. I will go to the gym and have a very intense workout, then the next day do a coffee enema, because it helps to draw the lactic acid out of the liver. Sometimes, I add in half a tablespoon of bicarbonate of soda [see Chapter 13] to help both with retention and to alkalise the body.

'From my research I knew that cancer cannot survive in an oxygen-rich environment and one which is alkaline. So my next step was to make my body as inhospitable as possible to cancer cells. I installed a proper water filter into my house, so all the water that we used for drinking and cooking was clean and free from chemicals, and I also used a water ioniser, which helps to make the water more alkaline. Shortly after my diagnosis I started taking a herbal tea called Flor-Essence which has anti-cancer properties (it is the original Canadian Essiac tea).

'I bought an ozone generator, from ozone expert Dr Saul Pressman in Canada, and self-administered ozone therapy both rectally and transdermally. I had also read about the benefits of far infrared sauna treatment, so I also invested in a small one-person unit. I combined the two therapies by heating up my body to a high level with the sauna and then, while still in the sauna, cupping the ozone to the site where the tumour was removed. The sauna kept my pores wide open while the ozone made its way in.

'Every morning I juiced organic carrots, organic celery and a green apple to which I added ground organic bitter apricot kernels, known for being the most concentrated source of B17. I followed the complete 'B17 Protocol' which includes pancreatic enzymes, zinc and several other supplements.

'In the afternoon I made fresh fruit smoothies, which included pineapple and papaya, because they contain some very potent anti-cancer enzymes – papain and bromelain. I also included some of the Brazilian super fruits – acai and acerola – which I bought frozen from a juice-bar supplier (you cannot buy them fresh). I cut out red meat and ate chicken and fish for protein.

'I supplemented with high doses of vitamins C and A, CoQ10, glutathione, alpha lipoic, selenium, shark cartilage, zinc, magnesium and several other supplements. I got back into exercise as soon as I could because that brings so many benefits both physically and mentally. That was six years ago – and looking back, the whole journey has been a blessing.

'Some people have questioned how I know for sure whether I'm cancer-free, since I have not returned to a hospital since my diagnosis. It might sound strange, and maybe even delusional, but I just know. Let me tell you why I took the decision not to go back – and I don't want anyone to think I am advocating this for them: I felt the stress of waiting for an appointment, which could be weeks or months, then waiting for the results, which again could be weeks, and finally hearing what the consultant has to say, was not worth the trauma. More importantly, what would they offer me if things had got worse? Chemotherapy, radiation or more surgery. How long can you keep cutting bits out and not actually addressing the root cause of the problem? The tumour is not the cancer; it is merely a symptom of the underlying problem. Fix the underlying problem or imbalance and the body will heal itself. I wanted to stay completely focused on what I was doing and more damaging radiation from scans, biopsies (known to spread cancer around) and the stress all of this puts on the body and mind, were not, I felt, conducive to my recovery plan.

'It is so important to take control and responsibility for your own health and educate yourself about the vast number of options available. Do not be bullied or pressurised into going down the conventional route – education is the key to success.'

Livia Casella, Australia: diagnosed 2007 – suspected melanoma

I tell this story to everyone. Black salve saved my life.

'The mole looked like a minuscule bunch of grapes, very small – maybe a centimetre in size. I went to the doctor and he said, "No worries Livia. It's nothing." But it was starting to itch like crazy – I knew something wasn't right.

'I showed it to a friend of mine, June, and she suggested I rub something called "black salve" on it. She said: "Look Livia, you have nothing to lose; if it's nothing, the black salve won't have any effect and if it's something more serious, the black salve will take it away." Within twenty-four hours of putting the paste on I could feel something happening. There was a very mild burning – a sort of drawing feeling. The next day the redness around the mole had gone from two centimetres to five.

'I decided to put the paste on again, this time all over the redness, not just on the little spot. Three days later I thought, Oh my God. This thing grew bigger and bigger. It looked like a spider with legs and I thought, Christ, what's going on? I didn't want to go to the doctor because I thought he would kill me for trying this "crazy" therapy.

'Thankfully, I had June to support me. I went to the chemist and bought a large gauze patch to cover the sore on my skin. At this stage, there was a pulling sensation and a bit of pain and I could see that something was coming out. I took some painkillers, so I wasn't so uncomfortable.

'By the fifth day this thing was the size of a dinner roll. It was like another breast. It was huge, painful, pusy and disgusting. It was monstrous. Then finally, it came off. It was like a piece of meat, red with roots – you had to see it. But after that? The pain disappeared.

'Interestingly, I hadn't been able to breathe properly for three years. I was constantly catching my breath and I didn't know why. But as soon as this "tumour" came off, I could breathe freely. I was told to put hydrogen peroxide [food-grade – see Chapter 9] on the wound on my chest. I did that three or four times a day and it wasn't painful at all.

'Three days later, you would not believe it! My breast had almost completely healed. Now all I have is a tiny white mark – as if I had had an operation and had stitches. It's minuscule. I could have lost two breasts and maybe my life, but instead I used the black salve for five days – and had three days of healing. I tell this story to everyone. It saved my life.

'We really wanted to get the "tumour" lab tested, so we took the specimen to the doctor, in a special hermetically sealed container, within hours of it coming off. But they said it wasn't "live" and they couldn't test it. What a joke!

'When I told my GP about what happened, he thought I was nuts. But to his credit he is actually now reading up about the black salve and told me a few months ago: "Well there's something here, I've got to admit it."

'A little while later, it was discovered that June's daughter-in-law had a skin cancer on the back of her hand. "Cutting into it would have damaged many nerves, so she tried the black salve which worked beautifully," says June. They went to the specialist, had tests done and she was cancer-free.'

Afterword

If you think black salve sounds medieval – you're right. Hildegard von Bingen, a gifted mystic, clairvoyant and healer, was said to have created it around AD 1100. The concoction is made from bloodroot, galangal root, zinc chloride and water. Although banned for use on humans in Australia (some believe this is purely profit driven), the fact is, anyone can make it. Holistic vets around the world use it to treat animals with certain cancers.

One of them is Dr Bruce Ferguson who is based at Murdoch University in Western Australia. 'When you apply it topically, it causes abnormal cells to necrose, or die,' Dr Ferguson explains. 'In a sense, it's better than a surgeon's eye, because a surgeon can't tell bad cells from good cells, but the black salve can,' he says.

Emil Brehm, Germany: diagnosed 2004, aged 64 – pancreatic cancer

... he remained convinced that the 'sugar tablets' would never cure a tumour like his.

As told by Emil's daughter, Patrizia Sergeant, who lives in the UK:

'In the summer of 2004 my dad was already showing symptoms: his urine was dark brown, his skin was incredibly itchy and at night he was waking up drenched in sweat. He then developed jaundice and weeks later, in September, he was diagnosed with pancreatic cancer.

'The doctors decided to go ahead with something called a Whipple procedure. This meant the removal of most of the pancreas together with a third of the stomach, gall bladder and duodenum. After the operation we were told that it had been unsuccessful; the tumour had grown around the aorta, which made it too dangerous to remove. We were told that my father's life expectancy was one year at the most and to enjoy every minute we had with him.

'It was hard to imagine that somebody as tough and strong as my dad could die of such a horrible disease. My father had never smoked or drunk too much alcohol, and had eaten a very healthy diet his whole life.

'One doctor offered a radical four-week programme of radio/chemotherapy to reduce the tumour, prior to carrying out another operation. I knew in my heart that wasn't going to help him, but I thought, I have to accept it because it's his body and his choice.

'But another doctor at the hospital in Germany said to us: "Careful when you're being advised to do chemotherapy or radiotherapy because it's for the statistics." He then added, "They can reduce the tumour – and that goes down in the statistics as a successful treatment. But how you die in the end? No one talks about that." He advised us to look into therapies from Eastern countries.

'I had heard about a successful homeopathic cancer treatment called the Plussing Method, developed by Dr Ramakrishnan, and I finally found a top consultant who is highly regarded in Germany, Dr Uwe Friedrich. He teaches at the Heidelberg University and has been practising homeopathy for thirty years. My dad respected him and immediately started taking the homeopathic remedies, although he remained convinced that the "sugar tablets" would never cure a tumour like his.

'Three months later Dad went to have his CT scan. While he was waiting a young doctor started chatting to him and asked, "What treatment are you doing? Are you doing chemo?" Dad said, "No, no. I'm doing homeopathy." The doctor started ridiculing my dad and said to him, "That's never going to get rid of it," then turned and walked away.

'Then Dad was called for his CT scan ... and the tumour was gone. When my mum told me, I thought she'd got it wrong. The doctors also thought they'd got it wrong; they thought the CT scan machine was broken. But the tumour *was* gone, and it never came back.

'But there was another aspect to Dad's cancer – and his recovery. He had never managed to enjoy his life and was always very tense. After his diagnosis he discovered – through doing a Brandon Bays Journey process with me – the root cause of his fears and anger – and, I believe, his cancer.

'The Journey process, in essence, is about releasing trapped emotions. With the help of someone trained in the process you uncover a stored memory linked to that unresolved emotion. Then you allow yourself to *feel* it fully, and the moment you feel it – it goes. It's incredibly liberating for many people and can lead to profound healing.

'During the process my dad went back to a time when he was two years old, when he watched his father beat up his mother. I said to him, "What do you feel?" and he said, "Fear." I'm sure recognising and releasing this trauma, which he'd held since he was two years old, has helped to keep the cancer away.'

Nicola Corcoran, UK: diagnosed 2010, aged 40 – stage-2 breast cancer

I changed everything that went in or on my body.

'It seems that there are two distinct periods of my life: Before Cancer and After Cancer. BC I was carefree and careless, fear-driven and disconnected. AC I am contented and present, motivated by love and constantly learning. But it can be lonely here. It takes a lot of effort to maintain health this way, and it's relentless. There's no ready-made network to tap into for support. There are no pink crowds running for me. However, it's important to understand that in everything we have choices. This is my choice, and one that I would make again and again. When I'm on top of it all – cooking each meal from scratch, juicing, meditating, supplementing and exercising – I feel amazing and invincible. But I'm not superwoman, and of course there are times when I feel overwhelmed and tired – when carrying this load feels like a heavy burden.

'I was diagnosed with invasive ductal carcinoma of the right breast (ER/PR positive, grade 2), onset of Paget's disease of the nipple and DCIS. One of thirty-two lymph nodes showed positive for disease. I had a mastectomy and, two weeks later, a full lymph clearance. Somewhere in between those two operations I started asking questions, and began taking responsibility for regaining my health.

'My husband and I were advised not to tell our children immediately. However, kids have an innate ability to sense when something is wrong, and in the absence of information, they came up with scenarios scarier than reality. Overnight, our house was filled with people – visitors crying and talking in whispers. It quickly became clear that our boys were feeling excluded and confused. We had always been open and honest with our children, so telling them wasn't difficult – maintaining a poker face was more challenging. We used child-friendly language, and kept it simple. We told them that I had found a lump and that it was called cancer. The doctor was going to take it out, and to do that he had to remove my breast. From that point on the conversations became child-led. Our eldest son was six years old, and told me that I mustn't be cross with the lump – I would make it angry, and it would grow (so wise). Our youngest was just three. I have no idea how you assimilate information like that at the age of three, but he gave it a good go. Lots of questions followed. Did it hurt? Was I scared? Would there be a big hole left in my chest after the operation? But they never asked me if I would die. The word "cancer" held no fear for my children because they had no negative associations attached to it.

'I quickly rejected chemotherapy, based on empirical evidence that there would (optimistically) be between a 5 and 12 per cent chance of it "mopping up" any micro-metastases. I later learned that chemo is great for de-bulking tumour mass, but it cannot destroy circulating cancer stem cells.

Instead, I looked to a good friend who is a naturopath for advice. She initiated what was to become a long and fascinating education in detoxifying and re-nutrifying my body. Initially my family was very concerned about my decision to reject allopathic medicine, but very quickly they came to trust and actively support me, particularly my husband.

'Interestingly, the lifestyle changes I've made have had an impact on the way that my immediate family and close friends think about their own health and nutrition. My husband fights me for time in the sauna, our sons are now gluten-free and as a family we eat only organic food. Friends have taken on board my lectures about cooking only with coconut oil, and my dad is treating his newly diagnosed diabetes solely with diet and nutrition.

I made big changes in small, manageable steps. The first change was to my diet. Although I'd been a vegetarian for over twenty-five years, I didn't understand about nutrition. Out went salt, sugar, gluten, dairy and alcohol. I bought a reverse osmosis ionising water filter and a juicer. I started putting lots of organic greens into my body and aided detoxification with coffee enemas, castor oil packs and Epsom salt baths.

'I changed everything that went in or on my body: make-up, deodorant, toothpaste, moisturiser and washing powder. I learned quickly how important it is to cook every meal from scratch: porridge, short-grain brown rice and salads are daily staples, along with nut milks, vegetable juices and green smoothies. I shifted my culinary focus away from a Western diet and started to get inspiration from Asia where dairy and meat are typically less important.

'Within a few weeks I began seeing a complementary doctor for high-dose vitamin C/hydrogen peroxide infusions with hyperthermia. I had preventative lymphatic drainage and acupuncture regularly and I also went to a holistic dentist and had my amalgam fillings replaced with clean composites. The UK charity Yes to Life gave me a grant to buy a far infrared sauna and I began practising yoga.

'I started to feel amazing!

'Next, I approached my emotional and mental health and

tried hypnotherapy, healing and reiki. Happiness lies in being present, and I now find myself observing situations and seeing what I can learn from them, rather than judging or using old behavioural responses. I say affirmations to myself daily – usually during a coffee enema. They sound something like this: "I am healthy, I am totally well" and "I love and approve of myself". It's important to really imagine yourself where you want to be, and to believe it to be true in this moment. Sometimes I feel resistance when I say one of the above affirmations, which is great because it shows me which areas need my attention.

'I also use visualisation techniques to imagine removing any residual cancer cells. Rather than "hunting and destroying" them, I take a kinder, gentler approach. I lie quietly in a meditative state and imagine any remaining cancer cells being neutralised by my body.

'Sleep is more important than I ever understood. In the period leading up to cancer, I was incredibly sleep deprived. My husband and I had struggled to conceive our sons and I was a fearful parent, overprotective and running to every nocturnal cry. For years I would wake up three times a night on average, and I was tired to the point of hallucinating. I was constantly unwell, but soldiered on with the help of a well-stocked medicine cabinet. Only when diagnosed with cancer did I magically find the time to look after myself and get enough sleep.

'I know now that the need to respect the body clock is far greater than our desire to reclaim some adult time in the evenings. The pineal gland waits for darkness before it starts to produce melatonin, and when we stay awake looking at the television or computer screen our pineal gland receives the message that it's still daytime. Even sleeping with a night light will disrupt our production of melatonin. This can eventually lead to a hormone imbalance. Oestrogen dominance is a strong precursor for certain cancers like prostate and breast. It has been proved that night-shift workers are more prone to breast cancer and, conversely, that blind women are less so. This is thought to be due to an excess of oestrogen and a lack of progesterone: a hormone imbalance linked to the suppression of melatonin production.

'The final piece of the puzzle was finding a functional doctor who is looking at my body's underlying weaknesses and rebalancing my system. I take natural hormone balancers (DIM, among others) and a range of supplements specific to my body's needs. In terms of screening I chose safer options: thermo-scans, rather than mammograms, and minimal residual disease testing [RGCC analysis, see Chapter 10]. I also had chemo-sensitivity testing to check which complementary medicines would have an impact on any circulating cancer stem cells which had spread into my body via the lymph.

'I continue to reject the one-size-fits-all approach to healing. I've learned incredible things over the past three years . . . things which have challenged the way I think and have altered the way I live my life. I no longer get ill, and many of the health issues I had prior to diagnosis (migraines, painful periods, candida, eczema, gum disease) have disappeared. I try not to be motivated by fear, but rather to live in the present, be guided by my intuition and understand that cancer has been an opportunity for me to become the person that I am today.

'My results, as of last week, show that my cancer stem-cell count is low and stable, essentially meaning that I have no evidence of disease and a low risk of metastasis. I can never go back to life BC, and I wouldn't choose to. I've learned far too much over the past three years to want to go back to being unconscious. In this new life there is more breathing, more laughing, more loving, more feeling. I am living with cancer, not dying of it, and I intend to carry on this way for many, many years to come.'

Nicola is author of the blog, Growing Through Cancer, www.growingthroughcancer.blogspot.co.uk

Jane Wallis, UK: diagnosed 2005, aged 59 – advanced bladder cancer

I used dowsing to 'ask' which people were beneficial to me, and who I should avoid.

'When I started getting up to go to the bathroom four times every night, I knew that something was up and I decided to go for a check-up. The doctors initially thought I had a prolapse of the bladder, since I had been doing heavy DIY work on my daughter's flat. While I waited for scans they put me on the waiting list for an incontinence clinic.

'Before the results came through I was seen by a young trainee doctor working in the hospital: she knew it was more serious. She did a manual feel and said she thought I had a tumour. But her diagnosis was dismissed after the scans came back negative. The supervising doctor said to me she was "only a trainee", implying that she didn't know what she was talking about. As I was leaving, a nurse who had witnessed this took my husband and me aside. In a whisper, she told us that her mother had had the same symptoms as me and was told there was nothing wrong, but she had died of cancer a few months later.

'Only when I started to haemorrhage lots of blood did the doctors agree that something was wrong, and after a camera inspection they found the cancer. It was rated T4 – the most virulent type according to the specialists – and it had gone right through the wall of the bladder to the fatty tissue beyond.

'The doctors told me the only answer was to have my bladder and most probably my kidney removed as this had also stopped working due to the tumour's location. On the same day I received the devastating news, we called in to see our good friend Dave on the way home. Dave – who was convinced that chemotherapy had killed his first wife – put some apricot kernels into my hand and said, "Here, these are what you need!" How right he was.

'My husband Nigel is a dowser and so we "asked" (using a pendulum) if the apricot kernels and other dietary changes I'd researched were going to be good for me and the answer was "Yes". I know many people believe that dowsing is all nonsense, but over the years I've found it incredibly helpful in many different areas. I also began to take Essiac tea, various vitamins and Chinese herbs and I started to follow the "pH Miracle" diet.

'Within what seemed like a few days my symptoms improved. So when the hospital contacted me to schedule my operation I told the surgeon's PA that I had decided against it and that I was going to treat the cancer myself. I will always remember the total silence that followed, before she put the phone down. A few minutes later she rang again to ask what I was doing before telling me she hoped I realised my cancer was really bad. I assured her that I understood, but this was my decision and that I would write to the surgeon to explain.

'A few days later I got a call from my local doctor asking me to come in and see him. He tried very hard to persuade me to have the surgery. As he was talking I glimpsed a copy of the letter I sent to the surgeon on his computer and saw that the surgeon had scrawled rude comments all over it. One remark that I remember vividly was: "Who does this bloody woman think she is?" When the doctor realised I could see the letter he switched the computer off very quickly. That was the last time I went in any doctor's surgery – over eight years ago. It only took eight months for my body to be 100 per cent cured after starting to take the apricot kernels and I've been well since then.

'My background in alternative healing no doubt informed the path I chose. I previously trained as a spiritual healer, and my teacher always said "cancer is the body's suicide note, and it will carry it out unless the person changes". She had noticed over many years that those who got better were the people who changed what was dysfunctional in their lives. So this really helped to give me strength to change what I knew I must. I now see my cancer as a kind of "temporary changing room"; somewhere where I "changed" by getting rid of all the toxins, situations and habits that I had to "take off" and leave behind.

'I knew I had to be careful what I took into my body – and not just food. Again, I used dowsing to "ask" which people were beneficial to me, and who I should avoid. I had always been too nice to tell certain friends that I didn't enjoy their company any more, but now when I found that their energies were not at all helpful, I was able to take responsibility and kindly tell them that I couldn't see them any more.

'My husband and I had both trained in shiatsu and worked with an energy master, so we know all about low vibrational energy, and how mobile phones and microwaves can emit harmful electromagnetic fields. Instead of having microwaved or frozen food, which I believe is missing vital energy, I concentrated on freshly cooked food and salads. I also knew it was important to remove any harsh chemicals – household cleaners and body products – so as not to stress the immune system when it was trying to heal.

'Watching the daily news, with the endless violence and problems, left me feeling depleted, so I decided to give that up too. I recently read a book called *Countdown to Coherence* by Hazel Courteney, a former *Times* columnist, in which she talks about being able to "smell" the stink coming from various newspaper articles and, indeed, from many parts of the man-made world. Now I make a conscious effort to "switch off" when I'm exposed to negative energy. I also believe having regular crystal energy therapy was vital for me.

'Certain books really helped me through this transformational process. Gregg Braden's *The Divine Matrix* taught me that the world is not as it seems – that it's jam-packed with the kind of miracles that the "white coats" might tell you are impossible. Other eye-opening books I read included *Dirty Medicine* by Martin Walker and *Quantum Healing* by Deepak Chopra. It was inspiring authors like these who showed me that real healing is possible, but you need to know and trust deep down that you will get better.

'I have never returned for follow-up scans, and when people ask, "How do you know that you still don't have cancer?" I reply, "I feel fantastic ... Why should I trust a scan to tell me I am now well when it couldn't tell me I was ill?" Unfortunately, I'm not the only one in my family who received a false negative from CT scans. My husband's sister was still being told, five weeks before she died of ovarian cancer, that her extreme pains were nothing serious – once again, it was only a physical examination by her GP that found the tumour.

'When I was first diagnosed I felt very much like Alice when she dropped down the rabbit hole, but very soon I started to see cancer as a blessing. It has taught me so many things and changed my life for the better, beyond anything I could ever imagine.'

Find Others in Your Shoes

Dr Kelly Turner has recently set up a research database of unexpected remission cases (www.unexpectedremission.org) where people can go to share their stories or seek inspiration. 'My goal is that a cancer patient could go to our research site and type in, "I am a female with stage-3 breast cancer, ER positive", and click a button that says: "Find me all the healing stories that match this." Then, rather than spend the night reading about what Herceptin is or what ER positive means, they could read twenty – maybe a hundred – stories of women just like them who had the same diagnosis and used other methods to get well.'

CHAPTER 13

Defeating Cancer on the Cheap

*'Good health makes a lot of sense, but
it doesn't make a lot of dollars.'*
Dr Andrew Saul, health educator and author,
in *Food Matters*

In Britain, Australia and the United States, you are punished financially if you choose alternative medicine over conventional treatment. Chemotherapy drugs are expensive – often tens of thousands of pounds[1] – but since they're covered by national or private health insurance, the patient usually pays only a small portion of that amount. Nevertheless, someone is footing the bill.

In 2011 Americans spent over $23 billion on cancer drugs.[2] Yet despite the promises, these shiny new drugs consistently under-deliver. 'Standard therapies, although free, condemn the patient to low survival rates,' says Dr Garry Gordon, co-founder of the American College for Advancement in Medicine (ACAM). 'Metastatic cancer five-year survival is 2.5 per cent;[3] alternative doctors prove 38–60 per cent [five-year survival] is possible.'

However, holistic medicine often comes with a hefty price tag. After just a few weeks of intravenous vitamin C injections, ozone therapy, and investing in a far infrared sauna, mum's credit card had already taken a battering. And that was before she flew to Germany for expensive blood tests. While mum has been lucky enough to be able to afford these things, for many people alternative cancer treatments can be financially crippling. 'It's okay for you,' people will say, 'but I don't have the money to see that specialist/order that supplement/travel overseas.'

Notwithstanding that money is a very real issue for a lot of people, there are effective solutions that don't cost the earth. In fact, some of the best things a cancer patient can do cost nothing at all. For Professor Jane Plant giving up dairy led to recovery. For Jane Wallis, a six-year bladder cancer survivor, apricot kernels and Essiac tea were, largely, the answer. 'In a cash market the first step in stopping cancer is diet,' emphasises Dr Garry Gordon. Giving up sugar – cancer's fertiliser – doesn't cost a penny, and filling up on green juices, although time-consuming, is relatively affordable – even if it means budgeting in other areas.

Getting out in nature and connecting with spirit is also free. How many of us have taken an early-morning walk on the beach and been soothed by the lapping waves? Or seen the sun go down over a mountain range and felt our body overcome with awe? Engaging with the natural environment bestows positive health benefits[4] and, in some instances, leads to profound healing. In *Peace, Love and Healing*, Dr Bernie Siegel discusses one case where Mother Nature contributed to a patient's 'spontaneous remission': 'Working outdoors, John maintains what I call a celestial connection and, like patients in the hospital who have shown to heal faster when their room has a view of the sky, he became healthier because of it.'

Changing your mental landscape can also change your life. Alternative cancer literature abounds with stories of tumours vanishing thanks to visualisation (Dr O. Carl Simonton, *Getting Well Again*), affirmation (Louise Hay, *You Can Heal Your Life*) and meditation (Ian Gawler, *You Can Conquer Cancer*). While these books remind us of what is possible, for many people it is simply incomprehensible to rely on non-tangible treatments to heal cancer. The large majority of people crave radical action in the face of a terrifying diagnosis.

So what *is* available for those on a budget? In researching this chapter I've learned that our world is rich in cancer-fighting substances. From broccoli sprouts and dandelion tea to shark cartilage and turkey-tail mushrooms there is a universe of affordable and effective options out there. However, I have decided to hone in on the five treatments that have consistently cropped up in the expert interviews, survivor stories and the medical research I've done:

- Marijuana

- Bicarbonate of soda

- Turmeric

- Salvestrols

- Homeopathy

And the phrase 'you get what you pay for' does not apply here; far from being maligned as 'poor man's treatments', these natural-health breakthroughs deserve to be part of anyone's healing arsenal, regardless of finances.

High on Healing

Cheryl Shuman was ready to die. After being diagnosed with advanced ovarian cancer, the celebrity, media and public relations expert was being treated with twenty-seven pharmaceutical drugs. 'I was basically a vegetable; I had a colostomy, a catheter, I couldn't go to the bathroom by myself,' Shuman divulged in a 2013 interview with American chat show queen Ricki Lake.[5] The tide turned, however, when Shuman started using alternative treatments, including cannabis oils and cannabis juices. Within ninety days, the Beverly Hills media executive was not only able to walk and talk again, but she was back at work, full-time. 'It [cannabis] saved my life, that's why I've dedicated the rest of my life to being an activist,' she said on the show.

Queen Victoria may not have been so outspoken, but she too reportedly used marijuana for menstrual cramps. In the nineteenth and early twentieth centuries Indian hemp, as it was then known, was often prescribed by doctors and written about in medical journals. In fact, Queen Victoria's physician, J. R. Reynolds, wrote a paper in one of the world's most prestigious journals, the *Lancet*, revealing that 'when pure and administered carefully, it [cannabis] is one of the most valuable medicines we possess'.[6]

Today marijuana is back in the news thanks to being recently legalised in several US States (at the time of writing, medical marijuana is legal in eighteen states[7]), but behind the scenes it's never really left the picture. This is particularly true with regard to cancer care. In 1990 44 per cent of oncologists surveyed (all members of the American Society of Clinical Oncology) said that they had already recommended cannabis to their patients and 54 per cent thought marijuana should be legally prescribable.[8] Most oncologists recommend cannabis to treat the side effects of chemotherapy and radiation, not the disease itself, but over twenty major studies have demonstrated that cannabinoids actually fight cancer directly.[9] 'It's been shown that cannabinoids arrest cancer growths of many different forms of cancer, including brain, melanoma and breast,' says author and physician Dr Mark Sircus: 'One literally has to be a fool not to consider using medical marijuana in one's cancer protocol after reading the research.'

In his e-book *Medical Marijuana*, Dr Sircus has put together a dizzying array of fully referenced medical data, pooled from leading universities and top oncological journals. In 2007 a Harvard Medical School study showed that marijuana cut lung cancer tumour growth in half;[10] in a 2002 study researchers in Madrid injected rats with the psycho-active compounds in marijuana and 'destroyed incurable brain cancer tumours';[11] and in 2010 the NBC ran a story with the headline 'Medical marijuana stops spread of breast cancer'. Summarising the research, Sircus writes: 'Cannabinoids offer front-line medicinal support for radiation exposure, cancer, diabetes and a host of neurological conditions. It is also the best and safest all-purpose pain medication ... Tetrahydrocannabinol [THC – the psycho-active component of pot] and natural cannabinoids counteract cancer and chemical toxicity from drugs and environmental sources thus helping to preserve normal cells.'

The first evidence of cannabis's anti-tumour potential was discovered by accident in 1974. A team of researchers at the Medical College of Virginia had been provided funds by the National Institutes of Health to find evidence that marijuana damages the immune system. Instead they found that THC 'slowed the growth of lung cancers, breast cancers and a virus-induced leukaemia'.[12] You might assume this groundbreaking revelation fuelled further research, but instead, the Virginia study was promptly shut down.

Stirring the pot

Despite the blackout from governments, the message that cannabis helps cancer patients is spreading like wildfire. David Hutchison, a British expat now living in Canada, came across the research when his sixteen-year-old daughter Beth was diagnosed with an aggressive form of brain cancer (glioma) in 2010. The hideous news could not have come at a worse time: Beth was diagnosed the same day David's wife was admitted to palliative care for end-stage breast cancer. Sadly, having exhausted all the avenues conventional cancer treatment had to offer, David's wife passed away.

David was determined to find another way for his daughter:

'I started researching and one of the first things I did was Google "glioma". I came to a Wikipedia page and under '"Treatments" I was surprised to see a mention of marijuana,' he recalls. The entry reads as follows: 'Cannabinoids may represent a new class of anticancer drugs that retard cancer growth, inhibit angiogenesis and the ... spreading of cancer cells.'[13]

His interest piqued, David contacted a friend, British neurosurgeon Dr Mansoor Foroughi, to find out more. 'I asked him, "Can you tell me Mansoor, am I chasing rainbows here: cannabis for a brain tumour?" and he said, "No, David, you're not chasing rainbows. I've got a paper about that; let me send you something."' In 2011 Dr Foroughi published a paper reporting on two children from Vancouver who experienced spontaneous regression of brain tumours. The report was published in the journal *Child's Nervous System*. In both cases, the tumour regression happened when the patients reached their early teens ... and started smoking marijuana. In the final conclusion the authors write: 'Further research may be appropriate to elucidate the increasingly recognised effect of cannabis/cannabinoids on gliomas.'[14]

With chemotherapy only offering Beth 'a little more time', David and his daughter decided cannabis was worth a try. In Canada medical marijuana is available through the National Health Service, and in 2011 Beth became the first child to be prescribed it by her neuro-oncologist. 'I hasten to say she's never smoked it,' says David. 'She started taking it in a cookie format, but now she takes it in a tiny oil capsule.'

From maple leaf to marijuana leaf?

Canada is a well-known hot spot for pro-cannabis supporters, perhaps none more famous than Rick Simpson, founder of Phoenix Tears. In 2003 Simpson successfully cured his own skin cancer with hemp oil and has recently published a book documenting his story – *Phoenix Tears: The Rick Simpson Story*. He has been providing people with instructions on how to make hemp oil medicines for about eight years: 'Hemp oil seems to work on all types of cancer and I am not aware of any type of cancer that it would not be effective for,' says Simpson whose website is packed with the latest research and real-life testimonials.

Unlike the standard cut, poison, burn procedures of conventional cancer treatments, cannabis will not damage healthy cells. So how does it work? 'When hemp oil is ingested as a cancer medication, the THC in the oil causes a build-up of a fat molecule called ceramide. When ceramide comes in contact with cancer cells it causes programmed cell death of the cancer cells while doing no harm to healthy cells,' explains Rick Simpson in a post in 2010.[15]

But for those who aren't thrilled at the idea of having to get high to heal cancer, there may be another option. Researchers from the University of Milan recently published a report concluding that the non psycho-active component – cannabidiol (CBD) – produces a significant anti-tumour activity both in vitro and in vivo. 'It's good for almost every medical situation, with or without the THC,' confirms Dr Mark Sircus, pointing to research in his book.

And it's safe for children too: 'When you're treating cancer and you're treating kids, it's the safest medicine – period,' says Dr Sircus. For Mike Hyde the side effects of conventional cancer care are all too real. After his two-year-old son Cash was diagnosed with stage-4 brain cancer he was subjected to seven different chemotherapy drugs. He subsequently suffered septic shock, a stroke and pulmonary haemorrhaging. According to a report on ABC news,[16] Cash was so sick he went forty days without eating and his organs were threatening to shut down. His father intervened, slipping cannabis oil into his son's feeding tube and Cash, who turned three in 2011, made a miraculous recovery.

Many ways to roll

While smoking a joint might be the most recognised delivery method, there are many other options: 'You can put it in food, you can juice it, you can put it in oil,' suggests Mark Sircus. 'With breast cancer ... it's very easy to be treated through the skin, so rubbing marijuana oil into the breast is great.' In her interview with Ricki Lake, Cheryl Shuman, also known as the 'Martha Stewart of Marijuana', shared her preference: inhaling cannabis oil through a special vaporiser,[17] similar to an electronic cigarette. Dr Sircus approves: 'It's a very ideal way of taking it because you don't have the toxic effect of burning the paper,' he says, adding that while smoking marijuana might damage lung cells, it has been shown to *prevent lung cancer*, an interesting anomaly uncovered by UCLA professor Donald Tashkin.[18]

With such a formidable body of research it's easy to believe that simply lighting up is all that's required to heal from cancer, *and for some, maybe it is*. But Dr Sircus cautions against throwing all the eggs into one basket: 'So topical marijuana, magnesium massages, sodium bicarb baths, handling emotional stress and learning to breathe properly are just some of the ways to increase our sense of certainty that the war on cancer can be won,' he says. In his book, *Treatment Essentials*, Dr Sircus outlines his full protocol for patients, based on a combination of low-cost treatments.

Bicarbonate of Soda

Before you scoff at the idea of using a cooking ingredient to overcome cancer, consider this: oncologists routinely administer bicarbonate of soda when they deliver chemotherapy.

I know. I was shocked too. According to Dr Sircus, sodium bicarbonate (also known as bicarbonate of soda and baking soda) is frequently used to keep the toxicity of chemotherapy agents and radiation from causing immediate harm to the patient: 'I always like to say, without the bicarbonate the chemotherapy will kill the patient on the spot,' says Dr Sircus. He discovered this by accident when he was combing through hundreds of medical papers in the process of researching his latest book, and came across a description of the nurses' protocol for administering chemotherapy agents. Bicarb is commonly used as an antacid for stomach upsets, as well as for gout flare-ups and urinary tract infections. This store-cupboard staple has also helped patients overcome diabetes, kidney problems and asthma, according to Dr Sircus.

The central argument for using bicarb for cancer is based on the idea of balancing the body's pH levels. 'It functions like bunker-buster bombs: it blasts cancer with shock waves of alkaline pH without harming the host,' expounds Sircus. In recent years 'alkaline' has become something of a buzzword among holistic health aficionados: we're told that Gwyneth Paltrow and Victoria Beckham are alkaline-diet devotees and that drinking 'Green Goddess' juice has something to do with it. But what does it all mean? 'If tissue pH deviates too far to the acid side, cellular metabolism will cease and oxygen deprivation will occur,' explains Dr Sircus. We now know that cancer favours a low-oxygen environment, but beyond keeping cancer at bay, an alkaline diet might also hold back the years: 'The alkaline way of eating is popular because it gives you clear skin, shiny hair, good nails – it's what happens on the inside. Your food is your medicine,' says Natasha Corrett, a vegetarian/alkaline chef and co-author of the best-selling *Honestly Healthy* cookbook.

Adding bicarb to an alkaline diet – think broccoli, garlic and olive oil – might fast-track your efforts to raise your pH. 'With bicarb, it doesn't have to take weeks, you can do it in a few days,' says Dr Sircus. And other cancer experts agree. Leading cancer specialist Dr Leonard Coldwell suggests taking a spoonful of bicarb with five spoonfuls of organic maple syrup, heated up to form a solid mass. The theory goes that this combination acts as a 'Trojan horse' since cancer cells will make a beeline for the syrup's high-sugar content and then be nixed by the baking soda. Dr Francisco Contreras offers bicarbonate therapy at his renowned Oasis of Hope clinic in Tijuana, Mexico: 'By increasing a cancer patient's body pH and making it more alkaline, alternative cancer treatments such as intravenous vitamin C and ozone therapy become much more effective,' he says.

Thousands of cancer patients credit Rome-based Dr Tullio Simoncini with saving their lives. The maverick doctor, who pioneered the use of bicarbonate of soda for cancer patients, believes all tumours are held together by a fungus and that bicarb is able to dissolve it. Dr Simoncini's standard protocol involves administering a diluted bicarb solution intravenously. Sometimes he may place catheters in certain arteries, to provide an infusion of bicarb directly to the tumour.

No standard recipe

Bicarbonate of soda is a versatile ingredient. You can add it to a green juice, nebulise it straight into your lungs, add it to enemas or dissolve it in water. The only rule you want to abide by is to purchase an *aluminium-free* brand: Vincent Crewe, now six years on from a diagnosis of metastatic colon cancer, uses Arm & Hammer; there is another premium brand called Bob's Red Mill, available in the UK, America and Australia. Incidentally, Arm & Hammer promoted the medical use of bicarb in a small booklet published by them in 1926.

For mum, a bicarb and magnesium bath has become a bi-weekly ritual. Dr Sircus recommends this for anyone who's feeling a bit run down: 'The very best treatment when one first notices a foul smell, foul taste or flu-like symptoms, is to jump into a bath with several pounds of bicarbonate and magnesium salts,' he says.

So is bicarb dangerous?

As with any natural substance (including water) you can overdo it. Pre-clinical studies show that too much bicarbonate of soda continued for too long will be harmful to normal tissues, especially kidney and bladder tissues. Dr Mark Sircus emphasises the importance of getting the dose right: 'The key to safe use of sodium bicarbonate is the monitoring and testing of both urinary and saliva pH with pH test paper or an electronic tester. I recommend people do this every morning and chart their results, and whenever taking strong baking soda baths, do the same thing soon after getting out of the tub. We do not want the urinary pH to go over 8.0, and Arm & Hammer suggests right on the box to stop therapy to let the pH drop back down after a week of high use,' says Sircus, adding that most cancer patients have very acidic body tissues pH around 4 or 5.[19]

The evidence

Studies from cancer treatment centres such as H. Lee Moffitt Cancer Center & Research and the Arizona Cancer Center have shown that oral bicarbonate therapy significantly reduces the incidence of cancer metastases in animal studies. In one 2009 study Dr Robert J. Gillies and his team reported that sodium bicarbonate raises tumour pH and inhibits spontaneous spread of cancer.[20] Galvanised by these results, Dr Gillies has initiated a formal clinical study evaluating sodium bicarbonate as a therapy for late-stage cancer patients.[21] He has also worked alongside researchers from Oxford and Bristol universities – with results published in the *British Journal of Cancer*.[22] In 2012 Dr Mark Pagel from the University of Arizona Cancer Center received a $2 million grant from the National Institutes of Health to study the effectiveness of bicarbonate of soda therapy to treat breast cancer.

Despite a hundred years of clinical use and research, some

claim that bicarb is no match for more established alternative cancer treatments like hyperthermia.[23] I am certainly not qualified to weigh in with my own opinion; I'm merely sharing with you the story so far.

As with any therapy, bicarb should be used in conjunction with a complete anti-cancer protocol. For further details see Dr Mark Sircus's book, *Sodium Bicarbonate – Rich Man's Poor Man's Cancer Treatment*.

Goodness Rising

Interestingly, when you take bicarbonate of soda it increases levels of CO_2 in the blood. It might sound counterintuitive, but increased levels of CO_2 actually mean increased levels of oxygen: 'CO_2 and oxygen are like a yin/yang pair, they go together. You increase one, the other goes up,' says Dr Mark Sircus. This is the reason bicarb is used as a leavening agent in baking. When moistened, it releases carbon dioxide, which causes cakes to rise. Athletes have also been known to use bicarb to lift their game, since it raises the oxygen-carrying capacity of the blood. It is this oxygen-boosting effect that makes it an ideal treatment for cancer (see Chapter 9).

The Golden Spice

Here is another anti-cancer hero you'll find in your pantry. It's used in sauces, mustards, pickles and curry powder. In India, a pinch of the spice is used to flavour almost every meal and provide dishes with a vivid yellow colour. I am, of course, talking about the knobbly root, turmeric.

Known as 'India gold', turmeric has been renowned as a healing powerhouse for thousands of years. In traditional Ayurvedic medicine, turmeric was used to help treat stomach upsets, liver problems, infectious diseases and gynaecological problems; it has also been shown to help relieve pain during labour, regulate the female reproductive system and purify the uterus and breast milk.[24]

Over the last two decades this folk remedy has undergone forensic analysis. Numerous animal studies have demonstrated turmeric's potential against neuro-degenerative diseases, depression, diabetes, obesity, atherosclerosis *and* cancer. In one study the active compound in turmeric reversed the growth of human breast cancer cells by 98 per cent.[25] In another it was shown to cause a 90 per cent reduction in cancers of the mouth and tongue caused by smoking.[26]

Professor Bharat Aggarwal, head of the Cytokine Research Group in the department of experimental therapeutics at MD Anderson, is a leading authority on the benefits of turmeric. The majority of cancer research has focused on a molecule called curcumin, which constitutes around 5 per cent of turmeric.[27] 'So far, nobody has found a cancer, at least in the test tube, that curcumin cannot stop,' says Professor Aggarwal. To date, the wonder molecule has proved its potential against colorectal, pancreatic, breast and prostate cancers, multiple myeloma, lung cancer, oral cancer, and head and neck squamous cell carcinoma.[28] 'You take any kind of cancer cell – it does the same thing,' confirms Professor Probal Banerjee, Professor of Neuroscience at the College of Staten Island, New York. Banerjee published a paper in 2009 showing that curcumin successfully blocks brain tumour formation.[29]

Both Banerjee and Aggarwal hail from India. 'Growing up, we would make a paste of turmeric and slaked lime and rub it on sprained ankles,' says Banerjee. 'We knew it was anti-inflammatory and anti-microbial; that's why people sauté vegetables, fish and meat in turmeric – it helps keep it from spoiling.' In India – producer and consumer of most of the world's turmeric – colon cancer rates are 'almost zero' according to Banerjee, and the incidence of prostate cancer is the lowest in the world. Figures from the International Agency for Research on Cancer reveal that a mere 5 out of 100,000 Indian men develop the disease annually, versus 125 out of 100,000 in the United States.[30] Coincidence? Professor Aggarwal doesn't think so. Alongside his team at MD Anderson, he has published over a hundred papers demonstrating the anti-cancer benefits of turmeric, and some of the results are astonishing. In one study, researchers found that curcumin blocked a biological pathway needed for the development of melanoma and other cancers – including prostate tumours. So impressed was Aggarwal that he coined the nickname 'cure-cumin'.

Despite hundreds of pre-clinical trials on animals, however, data on humans is relatively sparse. 'We have a very big problem with funding,' explains Aggarwal. 'Most clinical trials are funded by pharmaceutical companies, and they aren't interested in turmeric because it can't be patented.' But that hasn't stopped patients streaming into Aggarwal's office. They don't have time to wait for phase-three clinical trials: they want this natural cure-all now. Over one thousand patients have sought out Aggarwal and started his curcumin regime (8 grams of curcumin/turmeric a day, spread out over four doses). Many of them felt moved to share their experiences online.[31] Sophie is one of them.[32]

Eight years ago Sophie was diagnosed with lymphoma. She arrived at MD Anderson and was told to start chemotherapy immediately. Aged thirty-five and the mother of two young children, Sophie asked whether she could wait for her mother-in-law to come to town, to help her get through the rigours of treatment. 'How long will that be?' the doctor asked. 'Three months,' she responded. The doctor decided it was okay to wait.

While visiting the hospital, Sophie ran into Professor Aggarwal and, after learning about curcumin, decided it was worth a shot. She began taking curcumin capsules twice a day, gradually escalating the dose until she was taking 8 grams. After three months she returned to MD Anderson and told the doctor she was ready to start chemo. But he wasn't. After examining her, the doctor apparently said: 'You don't have cancer. You don't need chemo. Just keep on doing whatever you're doing, but I don't want to know about it.'

For the next five years Sophie continued taking the curcumin capsules and having six-monthly check-ups. The scans continued to show no sign of cancer; that is, until she decided to scale back her daily dose. Sophie went from taking 8 grams of curcumin a day to 4 grams – and with that, the cancer came back. But when she returned to taking 8 grams a day? The cancer went away. 'So what did that mean?' says Aggarwal. 'Curcumin made the cancer quiet; it made her lead a normal life, where nobody is causing any trouble for her and everyone is happy.'

So how does curcumin work?

Unlike conventional cancer treatment, which indiscriminately kills fast-growing cells in an attempt to get to the cancer, curcumin *selectively* kills cancer cells. 'There is no drug available, that can selectively go after the bad guy, but curcumin does that,' says Aggarwal. The FDA has published a 200-page report on the safety of curcumin and it has been given the label GRAS – meaning generally regarded as safe.

But this is far from a mild home remedy. The latest research shows that curcumin has the power to tackle cancer at its source; it can wipe out cancer stem cells. All too often, these slow-growing cells are left behind following standard treatment and, according to experts, are the reason why cancer comes back. Professor Banerjee explains that this is particularly pertinent to gliobastoma, a highly resistant form of brain cancer. 'The standard procedure for this cancer is surgery, radiation and chemo-therapy – but so often it will come back,' says Professor Banerjee. 'The main reason is that chemotherapy only goes after the fast-dividing cells, and what's left behind are the cancer stem cells which grow very slowly.' Banerjee has found that by attaching curcumin molecules to specific antibodies he is able to target the stem cells and 'blast off the tumour' in mice.

Nutritional chemotherapy

When you combine turmeric with black pepper it multiplies the effectiveness by 1000 times, according to Ty Bollinger, author of *Cancer: Step Outside The Box*: 'It makes the most powerful "natural chemotherapy" you can ever experience,'[33] he writes, adding that curcumin can also protect cells against oestrogen-mimicking chemicals. This is the same mechanism by which the popular breast cancer drug Tamoxifen works. However, this hormone-blocking therapy has its drawbacks. It has been repeatedly shown to increase the risk of liver cancer and double the risk of endome-trial cancer.[34] While no experts have suggested that turmeric could replace Tamoxifen, the research is tantalising. Turmeric can also protect against the damage caused by radiation[35] and boost levels of that all-important antioxidant glutathione (see Chapter 5).

After learning about its benefits, mum started adding the golden root to her daily juice. She also now eats curry regularly (it has replaced spaghetti as the comfort food of choice) and she occasionally treats herself to a chocolate and turmeric face mask (very anti-ageing, according to skin guru Dr Nicholas Perricone[36]). When I quizzed Banerjee about mum's self-styled protocol he gave juicing the green light: 'When you juice it [whole turmeric], it goes into your stomach and interacts with surfactants which will emulsify the curcumin and make it more soluble.'

For those who can't get hold of the fresh turmeric root (it looks like a cross between ginger and galangal) there is a huge range of supplements available. Professor Banerjee recommends a product called Curamin, which contains a special form of curcumin called BCM-95®. 'It's basically nano-curcumin. You can go very high on that – 12 grams a day without any problem at all.' According to research from the Curamin website, the product has up to ten times more bioavailability than standard curcumin extracts.

You might assume that if you're dealing with something like cancer, it's better to flood your body with as much turmeric as possible, but according to Professor Aggarwal, people should start low. He encourages patients to start with 500 milligrams and gradually increase the dose to 8 grams, if required. For those who are considering taking turmeric alongside chemotherapy, Professor Aggarwal points to pre-clinical studies showing that curcumin enhances the effect of most chemotherapeutic agents including Velcade, Revlimid, cisplatin, 5FU, doxorubicin and others.[37] However, as with everything, we recommend consulting your supervising physician.

Salvestrols

Is organic really better? While academics continue to argue the point, cancer survivors are living proof that eating organic food can help send cancer packing. In 2012 the *Telegraph* newspaper in the UK published a feature about the Marchioness of Worcester, who credited an organic diet and complementary medicine with helping her beat breast cancer.[38] 'I am almost religious about it now,' she said. All over the internet you'll find similar testimonies from survivors who swear up and down that organic is the only way. It certainly makes logical sense to reduce the body's toxic burden in order for it to heal. Research has also shown that organic fruits and veggies have up to 50–60 per cent higher levels of nutrients.

These factors alone should be enough to convince anyone to make the switch to organic, but for those who still aren't buying it, consider this: scientists have discovered certain plant compounds can induce cancer cell death, and these compounds have been shown to be 30 per cent higher in organic foods.[39] Described as 'salvestrols', these chemicals release a stream of cancer-killing agents when they come into contact with an enzyme found in cancer cells called CYP1B1 (pronounced 'sip one bee one').

Salvestrols are part of a plant's natural defence system. Fruits, vegetables and herbs produce them in order to repel bugs and pathogens. 'So when a plant is exposed to, say, fungi it produces compounds that are, in essence, anti-fungal,' says leading nutritionist Patrick Holford. 'These compounds we collectively call salvestrols. But if you spray a plant with fungicides, it won't produce salvestrols; it's as simple as that.'

Where 'salvestrols' sprouted

British pharmacologist Professor Dan Burke was the first to identify the enzyme CYP1B1 in 1995. He subsequently teamed up with Gerry Potter, Professor of Medicinal Chemistry at Leicester's De Montfort University, to investigate further. Together, the British professors were in the process of developing a synthetic pharmaceutical drug based on the groundbreaking discovery when they stumbled upon something remarkable: the compounds they were looking for already existed in nature. 'Gerry Potter discovered that when compounds which he called salvestrols come into contact with this enzyme, they selectively kill cancer cells,' says Holford. 'Because salvestrols are activated only within cancer cells, they offer the possibility of anti-cancer treatment without the horrible side effects.'

So how potent are these plant chemicals? Danica Collins, editor of *Underground Health Reporter*[40] is willing to put some heft behind them: 'When taken daily, salvestrols can kill clusters of cancer cells at a time ... prevent cancer cells from turning into full-blown, aggressive cancer ... and treat pre-cancerous cells containing the CYP1B1 enzymes,' she writes, adding that they act quickly and their effects last from three to ten hours.

The best part? You don't need to spend a fortune on exotic berries – apples are a good source of these anti-cancer agents. But choose carefully. 'Pendragon apples, which are rather hard to come by, have the highest salvestrol effect,[41] Cox apples are also pretty good and Gala apples are pretty useless,' clarifies Holford. As a general rule, bitter foods tend to contain more salvestrols, but it's difficult to accurately rank foods in order of potency, since that will vary according to where (and how) they are grown. Broadly speaking though, organic broccoli, grapes and parsley are high in salvestrols – indeed 'green and red' fruits and vegetables are the way to go, according to Professor Potter.

So how many salvestrols do you need to stay healthy? According to Holford, it will take more than just your 'five a day'. He estimates that a non-organic diet will deliver twenty points a day, if you eat five or more portions, while an organic diet will yield sixty to seventy – still short of the 100 points needed to stay healthy and nowhere near the amount required to overcome serious illness.

For those facing cancer, Holford typically recommends a 2000-point dose of salvestrols twice a day, but he urges people to seek personalised guidance from a qualified nutritional therapist. While the evaluation of salvestrols is ongoing, research is moving slowly. Like curcumin, salvestrols are natural compounds which cannot be patented – ergo, the funding is not available to conduct clinical trials. However, five encouraging case reports have been published in the *Journal of Orthomolecular Medicine*. These included patients with various-stage cancers of the lung, melanoma, prostate, breast and bladder. 'In all cases the response was positive and for some apparently curative,' says Holford.

'So will it work for me?' Frustratingly, there is no definitive answer to that ever-tempting question. But Holford offers some thoughts: 'My view, which is borne more out of logic than out of proven clinical trials, would be that if you took a period of three months and flooded the system with salvestrols and vitamin C, you are going to certainly give cancer cells a very hard time to survive ... while you do whatever else you do, be it conventional or alternative, or improving your diet as lifestyle as well.'

Homeopathy

Next time somebody gives you a ribbing for rubbing Arnica on a bruise or knocking back Ferrum Phos at the first sign of a flu, you might want to mention this: research has shown homeopathy works as well as an expensive breast cancer drug. In the study, published in the February 2010 issue of the *International Journal of Oncology*,[42] researchers at MD Anderson found the cancer-killing effects of four homeopathic remedies showed similar activity to Taxol, a commonly used chemotherapeutic drug for breast cancer – but without the toxic side effects on healthy cells. I spoke to the lead author of the study, Dr Moshe Frenkel, who is now based in Israel where he is the founder and director of Integrative Oncology Consultants:[43] 'The response from around the world was tremendous,' he says, 'but there were obviously critics ... '

Homeopathy is, without a doubt, mainstream medicine's favourite whipping boy. Doctors call it 'hocus pocus' and 'worse than witchcraft' and yet the National Cancer Institute in America, following an exhaustive evaluation,[44] concluded that there was sufficient evidence of efficacy to support further research. The controversial technique is centred on the idea that the symptoms of illness – say a fever or runny nose – are the body's attempts to heal itself. Therefore, a substance which can cause these 'disease-like symptoms' is given to patients to stimulate their immune system. Leading naturopath Val Allen uses the metaphor of vaccinations to help us understand:

'With vaccinations you're introducing a tiny amount of something noxious, like a disease, into a person, so their immune system creates antibodies to that particular substance and that person gains immunity to it. When you're looking at homeopathy, we're trying to trigger a similar response in the body, by introducing a very tiny harmless amount of that substance, so the body makes its own appropriate responses to that,' says Allen.

It is these 'harmless amounts' that conventional medicine finds it difficult to understand – many of the homeopathic doses are diluted thousands of times, to the point where no molecule of the original substance remains. It may defy the law of [current] physics, but somehow it works – at least, that's the conclusion people the world over have come to. From Southern India to South America,[45] people are using these tinctures – not just for sore throats and period pain, but for serious illness. One questionnaire-based study showed that homeopathy was one of the eight most popular complementary therapies used by cancer patients in the UK,[46] while a study in an oncology department in France in 2007 found that 34 per cent of patients were using complementary medicine and that among those patients homeopathy was the most frequently used.[47] The results from a survey at two oncology day hospitals in Italy found that 17 per cent of patients used CAM, with herbal medicine and homeopathy, again, being the most popular.[48]

In India, homeopathy – which bears similar traits to traditional Ayurvedic medicine – is widely accepted. 'Of course, homeopathy is much cheaper – ten times cheaper – than allopathic drugs,' says Dr Probal Banerjee. 'I grew up on homeopathy; I still use homeopathy – because of my mother.' Dr Banerjee's mother, a trained doctor, used to distribute medicine to the people free of charge. She was also a homeopath. 'My mother had treated and cured people with melanoma in India using homeopathy,' says Banerjee, who still uses it at the first sign of a cold (Dulca Mara 30x) and, when living in Bangalore, he regularly relieved visiting professors of severe diarrhoea with one homeopathic dose (Carbo Veg 6x or 3x).

As a family physician, Dr Moshe Frenkel had also seen homeopathy work in a variety of situations, but he never considered it a possible treatment for cancer. That is, until he worked at MD Anderson. 'I used to sit with patients for long periods of time – sometimes two hours – and I heard fascinating stories,' says Frenkel. 'Usually physicians are concentrating on following their guidelines and sometimes they forget that the patient might have a different agenda or different questions.' Dr Frenkel would come in with a blank canvas: 'I would ask them, "What are your concerns and how do you want me to address those concerns?"' says Frenkel. One of the things that came up was the use of homeopathic remedies.

Spurred on by his patients' interest, Frenkel decided to investigate further. He contacted a colleague, Dr Sen Pathak, professor of cell biology and genetics, who had conducted a number of trials alongside a hospital in India. In one of the trials, fifteen patients with brain tumours were given two homeopathic remedies (Ruta 6 and Calcarea Phosphorica 3x). Six of the seven patients with gliomas had complete regression.[49] Commenting on the study, Bryan Hubbard, publisher of *What Doctors Don't Tell You*, says: 'The result is astonishing. Gliomas are considered to be incurable; of 10,000 people diagnosed with malignant gliomas each year in the US alone, only around half are alive a year later, and just 25 per cent two years later.'

Dr Frenkel was similarly moved – so much so that he decided

to travel to India to visit the Prasanta Banerji Homeopathic Research Foundation (PBHRF) where the trial took place. Headed up by Dr Pratak Banerji and his son, Dr Pratip Banerji, the clinic has been testing homeopathic remedies on cancer patients since 1992 and they now treat around 120 patients every day.

'I saw things there that I couldn't explain,' says Dr Frenkel. 'Tumours shrank with nothing else other than homeopathic remedies ... X-ray showing there is a lesion on the lung and a year after taking the remedy it has shrunk or disappeared.'

As documented by the clinic, over 20,000 patients with malignant tumours were treated only with the Banerji protocol between 1990 and 2005. In 19 per cent of the patients, the tumours completely regressed, and in 21 per cent the tumours were stable or improved with treatment.[50] Bryan Hubbard sheds light on these figures: 'This suggests that homeopathic remedies on their own are reversing, or certainly stabilising 40 per cent of all cancers, a success rate that matches the best results for conventional medicine, and without the debilitating side effects of chemotherapy and radiation.'

Dr Frenkel stresses that the treatments did not work for everyone, but he believed the non-toxic treatment merited further study. On returning to MD Anderson Dr Frenkel got together a team of distinguished researchers to test the value of four ultra-diluted remedies against breast cancer cells. 'I asked my colleagues to look at the remedies as if they were the newest chemotherapy ... using the same framework they would for any new drug they would want to put into the market,' says Frenkel. When the initial results came in that the remedies selectively killed cancer cells, one of Frenkel's colleagues demanded a retrial. 'So he [the colleague] managed to get another lab in MD Anderson, a completely different lab, to run the trial again. And they got the same result.'

Despite the rigours of the study, many still questioned the paper. In response to the criticism, Dr Frenkel encouraged his peers to repeat the experiment. 'I said to them, "If you come to a different conclusion then why not publish a paper saying it doesn't work?"' Tellingly, not one of the scientists took up the challenge. Although the National Cancer Institute has declared an interest in Dr Banerji's protocol (after he brought them pathology reports and CT scans from exceptional patients) nothing has materialised. 'We're in a stuck situation right now,' says Frenkel, adding that, as ever, funding is a 'major issue'. 'Homeopathic remedies are cheap; they are a few dollars,' says Frenkel. 'So there are no drug companies who would make a lot of money out of them.'

Homeopathy became part of mum's anti-cancer regime when she returned from Germany. She tried to get hold of mistletoe (typically administered by subcutaneous injection) after molecular blood analysis revealed it was the best immune-boosting supplement for her. Failing to source the substance, mum had just about given up on the idea when her naturopath Val Allen found a solution: 'We're allowed to use mistletoe homeopathically,' says Allen who has combined the mistletoe extract (Viscum album) with two other immune-boosting extracts. 'While they look like tiny amounts of substances, they are quite profound in providing a base information profile for the immune system to create healthy, strong cells with a resistance to cancer,' says Allen.

As with any therapy, alternative or otherwise, it's vital to do your research and a find a practitioner who is not only experienced in their field, but also knowledgeable about *your* condition.

Time for Change

As an integrative oncology consultant, Dr Moshe Frenkel is able to offer patients valuable advice on homeopathy and other holistic therapies, and how they might enhance other chosen treatments (conventional or otherwise). Dr Frenkel takes pains to stress that one line of treatment is rarely enough. 'You can't just do one thing and ignore the others,' he says, citing the significance of exercise, stress reduction and nutrition. He also emphasises the importance of a patient's attitude.

Dr Frenkel explains that he recently conducted a study with MD Anderson looking at exceptional patients[51] – survivors who became disease-free or experienced unexplained survival time after being told their condition was terminal. The study revealed that 'patient activism' was a major theme. This found expression in various ways, including playing an active role in the choice of treatment and physician. According to the report, in many cases this involved 'an active process of data collection, examining the various physicians and seeking a second opinion'. Interestingly, when I asked leading oncologist and hyperthermia expert Dr Herzog if he had any recommendations for cancer patients on a budget, he said: 'They should try to get a second opinion, that's always important.'

Taking an active role in your health might require energy and willpower, but it doesn't cost a dime. In Dr Frenkel's report many exceptional patients made the conscious choice to view – and live – life differently, following their diagnosis. In some cases it was as simple as 'doing things I love' or 'becoming a little bit more self-centred'. While not everybody has the cash to spend on expensive treatments, all of us can afford some small change. However, if we want to collectively reverse the current cancer statistics, transformation is required on a grander scale. Not just personally, but politically. Cancer plays a significant role in the rising cost of healthcare – yet we are making little progress. America's National Institutes of Health has predicted that spending on all cancer treatment will rise from $125 billion (spending for 2010) to at least $158 billion in 2020. When Britain's National Institute for Health and Care Excellence (NICE) rejected several new cancer drugs the public was so outraged that the

British government did a U-turn and created a separate fund to pay for expensive oncology drugs. What if there were safer, cheaper, more effective alternatives? What if these could be used alongside expensive conventional treatments to enhance results? I'll leave you with that thought.

Epilogue

think my twenty-ninth birthday will remain the best birthday of my life. I woke up to the sun beaming through the shutters of my sister's old bedroom in Perth. I sat on the balcony and meditated to the sound of the galahs singing in the Tipuana tree and thought, How lucky am I: my mum is in the next room, she's healthy and the beach is calling our name. But before I answered that call I checked my email and discovered that I'd been offered a book deal. It was the cherry on the cake, the silver lining to a tumultuous journey that mum and I had embarked on following her diagnosis of cancer and during which I'd started writing a blog about her experience.

In blazing her own path mum has taught me so many valuable lessons: that it's worth standing up for what you believe in, that cancer can be a teacher as much as an enemy, and that finding a sense of meaning amid the injustice of illness is all-important if you want to heal. She has also shown me that healing from cancer is hard work. I admire the way she has stuck with her regime – from braving the pungent Haelan drink every morning to taking the coffee enema kit away with her on holiday – changed the way she responds to stressful situations and given up things that she loved in order to put herself on the road to recovery.

Taking responsibility for your health is by no means choosing the easy way out, but the results are often worth the effort. Many survivors I've interviewed in the course of writing this book have spoken of the satisfaction gained from personally uncovering the elements that were sabotaging their health and finding the missing pieces of their healing puzzle.

I have cried many times in writing this book – at the horror of young lives derailed by disease and in frustration at the red tape denying patients access to life-saving treatment. But I have also been comforted with the knowledge that our bodies and minds are so much more powerful than we think, and that there are passionate physicians willing to step outside the box – and even put their careers on the line – for their patients.

While I hope this book has brought you important information, nothing compares to the innate intelligence of your own intuition. What resonates with you? How does your body feel when you take a supplement or try a new therapy? Are these things you can discuss with your physician and if not, what's stopping you from finding a doctor who's on the same page as you? The idea that 'cancer is not a one-size-fits-all disease' cannot be emphasised enough: what works for one person might not work for the next. However, there are time-honoured tonics that anyone can benefit from – gratitude, oxygen and sunshine, to name a few – while forgiveness, physical activity and doing something that makes you lose track of time can also speed up your return to health.

It might seem simplistic to talk of these things when you're faced with cancer, and I'm certainly not inferring that they are all you need to make a full recovery. Cutting-edge treatments like hyperthermia and intravenous vitamin C or even conventional medicine might be more appropriate before you can even contemplate addressing the more esoteric things like emotional well-being. But whatever path you choose, don't ignore the fundamental aspects of good health: 'Every patient suffering with cancer I have seen did not begin to recover until they had addressed their emotional issues,' says Dr Rashid A. Buttar in *The 9 Steps to Keep the Doctor Away*.

Cancer is complicated. When you (or someone you love) are

first diagnosed it can feel like you're cramming for an exam: you quickly school up on terms like apoptosis, natural killer cells and mitochondria, while simultaneously trying to understand what drives cancer and remember which beauty products, light bulbs and dental fillings are the least carcinogenic. At first, the avalanche of information seemed overwhelming to me, but I realised quite quickly that it boiled down to a few key principles: get on top of stress and cut down on sugar; flood the body with oxygen and pull out the poisons; and put your faith in healing and fear behind you.

Fully understanding your condition and your treatment options is vital if you want to overcome cancer. When mum was first diagnosed we read countless books and spoke to a panel of experts before she started implementing her recovery plan. What we discovered is that education is as important as medication. 'The old meaning of physician was educator, and that is largely the role that I feel my staff and I should be filling for patients as we attempt to assist them in helping themselves,' says Dr Garry Gordon. David J. Getoff, who feels the same, suggests that when a person is first diagnosed they should purchase four or five DVDs on cancer therapies and watch them with a loved one.

In the wake of mum's diagnosis we embarked on something of a movie marathon. We'd snuggle up on her bed with a notebook ready and be awestruck and horrified in equal measure by the remarkable survivor stories and the financial agenda that underpins mainstream medicine. In the first few weeks we flew through the must-watch *CANCER is Curable NOW*, *Medical Renaissance: The Secret Code* (the celluloid equivalent of being wrapped in a warm, toasty towel), *Burzynski: The Movie* (about a Texan doctor curing universally fatal brain tumours) and Kris Carr's uplifting *Crazy, Sexy Cancer*.

Those first few weeks following a diagnosis of cancer are pretty grim. Life as you know it has been taken away and part of moving on means allowing yourself time to mourn. After one particularly trying weekend I remember mum saying, 'Is this it? Is this what my life is going to be like now?' Before she'd started to heal, and before we'd discovered just how many options were out there, it all seemed a bit hopeless. But then we started to watch, to read, to listen – and after a while, if we were very still, we could almost feel the hope trickle in.

The aim of this book is not to provide all the answers, but to raise your spirits along with a few important questions you might not otherwise have asked. Whatever road you decide to take, it's been a privilege to be with you on your journey, and I hope I've given you some comfort along the way.

Ten Golden Rules to Remember

1. You are not a helpless victim of your genes.

2. Your emotions matter more than you think.

3. Knowledge is power; do your research, then choose what feels right for you.

4. Follow your intuition – it's your body talking.

5. Play detective: is there an element you've overlooked that is sabotaging your health?

6. Remember, cancer loves sugar.

7. Detox: pull out the poisons and give your body the best chance of healing.

8. Find a doctor you respect and who respects you.

9. Work *with* your body, not against it.

10. Where attention goes, energy flows: fill your mind with stories of survivors; if they can do it, why not you?

On Love and Loss

Recently mum was at a funeral; one of the terrible ones. A bright future had been snatched away and a family was left grieving, forever changed. There are no words for these kinds of deaths, no comfort to quell the frustrated, angry, despairing sobs that leave you exhausted and utterly drained.

But the priest tried. He shared the following observation, taken from the *Tibetan Book of the Dead*:

'Almost all babies cry when they are born – and they come into a room full of people who are really happy. And then, when we die, most people look very peaceful and everyone around them is sobbing. Perhaps what we can deduce from this, is that we are very sad to leave the afterlife and very happy to return to it.'

Ultimately, we all return to Mother Earth, back to the ground that gave and gives us life. And yet, we never know – notwithstanding wheatgrass, yoga or prayer – when the time will come when we'll be forced to say goodbye to our families. But we can choose to live life full of love rather than fear – and sometimes death reminds us of that. 'Facing up to death can be the catalyst for the kind of profound internal change that allows us to love, often for the first time in our lives,' writes Dr Bernie Siegel.[1]

Notes

Introduction

1. National Cancer Institute: Surveillance Epidemiology and End Results (SEER), Cancer Statistics Review, http://seer.cancer.gov/statfacts/html/ all.html.
2. Emery, G., 'Are cancer patients' hopes for chemo too high?' Reuters, 24 October 2012; http://bit.ly/TfRSso, *New England Journal of Medicine*, 25 October 2012.

Chapter 1

1. McKillop, W. J., et al., 'The use of expert surrogates to evaluate clinical trials in non-small cell lung cancer', *British Journal of Cancer*, 1986, 54, pp. 661–7; http://www.whale.to/cancer/benjamin2.html; Day, P., *Cancer: Why we're still dying to know the truth*, Credence Publications, 2000.
2. http://panacea-bocaf.org/alternativecancertreatments.htm; http://www.naturalnews.com/023663_cancer_family_WHO.html#i xzz2Jjml91Iw.
3. www.reuters.com/article/2009/03/10/us-cancer-ovarian-idUSTRE 52974Y20090310.
4. Anderson, M., *Healing Cancer From the Inside Out*, Ravediet.com, 2008.
5. Moss, R. W., *Questioning Chemotherapy*, Equinox Press, 1995 (p. 8).
6. Cairns, J., 'The treatment of diseases and the war against cancer', *Scientific American*, 1985, 253, pp. 51–9.
7. www.ncepod.org.uk/2008report3/Downloads/SACT_report.pdf# search='chemotherapy; www.abc.net.au/news/2008-11-13/chemo therapy-contributes-to-a-quarter-of-cancer/204358.
8. American Cancer Society's (11th) Science Writers' Seminar, 28 March–2 April 1969, in which he confirmed what he had written as early as 1955, in his classic paper 'Demographic Consideration

of the Cancer Problem', published in *Transactions of the New York Academy of Sciences*, series II, vol. 18, pp. 298–333.

9. Dubner, S. J. and Levitt, S. D., *SuperFreakonomics*, Penguin Books, 2009 (pp. 85–6).

10. www.forbes.com/sites/gerganakoleva/2012/04/30/dr-otis-brawley-says-health-care-talk-in-u-s-lacks-human-element/.

11. www.macmillan.org.uk/Documents/AboutUs/Research/Research andevaluationreports/LivingAfterCancerMedianCancerSurvival Times pdf.

12. Quote from Dr Garry Gordon: 'DCIS (Ductal Carcinoma in-situ), is *not* a true Cancer. It is just a pre-cancer condition and, as such, these patients do *not need* radical surgery, chemo, or radiation.'

13. Herring, J., 'Three Proven Ways to Survive Cancer (and Chemo-therapy)', *Natural Health Dossier*, August 2012, issue 28, p. 3.

14. Spreen, A., *Tomorrow's Cancer Cures Today*, Health Sciences Institute, 2009 (p. 9); http://curezone.com/art/read.asp?ID=91&db =5&CO= 779.

15. 'Newton-John hopefully devoted to wellbeing', *The Australian*, 17 March 2007, www.news.com.au/news/newton-john-hopefully-devoted-to-wellbeing/story-fna7dq6e-1111113168397.

16. Moss, R. W., *Questioning Chemotherapy*, Equinox Press, 1995 (p. 35).

17. McTaggart, L. *The Bond*, Hay House, 2011 (p. xxiv).

18. Dubner, S. J. and Levitt, S. D., *SuperFreakonomics*, Penguin Books, 2009 (p. 84).

19. Herring, J., 'Three Proven Ways to Survive Cancer (and Chemotherapy)', *Natural Health Dossier*, August 2012, issue 28, p. 3.

20. www.huffingtonpost.co.uk/2012/08/06/health-chemotherapy-backfire-boost-cancer_n_1745856.html.

21. *Nature Medicine*, 2012, 18, pp. 1359–68, www.nature.com/nm/journal/v18/n9/fig_tab/nm.2890_F2.html.

22. www.greenmedinfo.com/blog/chemo-and-radiation-actually-make-cancer-more-malignant.

23. http://wn.com/professor_max_wicha__breast_cancer_stem_cell_ regulation; Ji, Sayer, 'Are Cancer Stem Cells the Key to Discovering a Cure?' 8 May 2012, Green Med Info (www.greenmedinfo.com/blog/are-cancer-stem-cells-key-discovering-cure).

24. Ibid.

25. www.ota.com/organic/mt/business.html.

Chapter 2

1. Quote from *Cancer Defeated!* newsletter, issue 182, http://cancer defeated.com/newsletters/The-doctor-who-cured%20too-many-patients.html.

2. Loyd, A. and Johnson, B., *The Healing Code*, Grand Central, 2011.
3. Sircus, M., *Medical Marijuana*, IMVA, 2012 (p. 15).
4. Paul, A. M., *Origins*, Hay House, 2010 (p. 46).
5. Siegel, B. *Peace, Love and Healing*, Rider, 1999 (p. 157).
6. *Science*, 2003, 302, pp. 643–50.
7. articles.mercola.com/sites/articles/archive/2012/06/13/keep-young-girls-away-from-xrays-as-new-study-shows-them-to-increase-breast-cancer-risk.aspx.
8. McTaggart, L., *The Bond*, Hay House, 2011 (p. 41).
9. *Cancer Genetics and Cytogenetics*, 15 April 2009,190 (2), pp. 81–7; PMID via www.greenmedinfo.com/print/blog/stress-hormones-found-make-cancer-resistant-treatment.
10. Moritz, A., *Cancer is Not a Disease – It's a Survival Mechanism*, Ener-chi Wellness Press, 2009.
11. Barasch, M. I., *The Healing Path*, Penguin Books, 1995 (p. 94).
12. I had the profound privilege of interviewing Andreas Moritz for this book before his life was sadly cut short. He helped people all over the globe restore their health and well-being; at the time of his death, Moritz had a two-year waiting list.
13. Siegel, B., *Peace, Love and Healing*, Rider, 1999 (p. 157).
14. Spiegel, D., et al., 'Effect of Psychosocial Treatment on Survival of Patients with Metastatic Breast Cancer', the *Lancet*, 1989, pp. 888–91.
15. Sircus, M., *Treatment Essentials*, IMVA, 2013.
16. www.cancersurvival.com/leshan.html.
17. Moritz, A., *Cancer is Not a Disease – It's a Survival Mechanism*, Ener-chi Wellness Press, 2009 (p. 128).
18. Palesh, O., et al., 'Stress history and breast cancer recurrence', *Journal of Psychomatic Research*, 2007, 63, pp. 233–9.
19. Turner, K., 'A Spontaneous Remission of Cancer: Theories from Healers, Physicians, and Cancer Survivors' (thesis submitted autumn 2010, University of California, Berkeley), p. 44.
20. www.dailymail.co.uk/health/article-198096/How-sleep-fight-cancer.html.
21. Siegel, B., *Peace, Love and Healing*, Rider, 1999 (p. 12).
22. usatoday30.usatoday.com/news/health/2005-03-21-stress_x.htm.

Chapter 3

1. Rossie, E. L., *The Psychobiology of Mind-Body Healing: New Concepts of Therapeutic Hypnosis*, W. W. Norton, 1986.
2. Study by psychiatrist Sandra Levy and Yale University psychologist Judith Rodin, reported in *Hippocrates*, November/December 1989, p. 93.

3. www.telegraph.co.uk/health/healthnews/7635143/Laughter-really-is-the-best-medicine-as-doctors-find-it-can-be-as-healthy-as-exercise.html.

4. Siegel, B., *Peace, Love and Healing*, Rider, 1999 (p. 28). (The primary factor was the length of time between diagnosis and cancer recurrence.)

5. undergroundhealthreporter.com/power-of-positive-thoughts#axzz2KUDDcmSC.

6. 'The survey of nearly 6,000 workers by the Chartered Management Institute found nearly half stay in contact with their employer while they are away', *Daily Mail*, 15 June 2005.

7. www.nytimes.com/2000/10/10/health/exercise-found-effective-against-depression.html.

8. http://www.ncbi.nlm.nih.gov/pubmed/15914748.

9. www.independent.co.uk/news/cancer-patients-too-polite-to-ask-for-best-treatment-1143265.html.

10. Plant, J., *Your Life in Your Hands*, Virgin Books, 2007.

11. Siegel, B., *Peace, Love and Healing*, Rider, 1999 (p. 27). (The study appeared in the *Lancet*.)

12. Ibid, p. 144.

13. Blyth Whiting, B., *Paiute Sorcery*, abridged in *Culture, Disease, and Healing Studies in Medical Anthropology*, ed. Landy, D., Macmillan, 1977 (p. 210).

14. Name changed.

15. Leith, W., 'How Anxious Are You?' *The Times Magazine*, 30 June 2012, www.thetimes.co.uk/tto/magazine/article3456097.ece.

16. Dr Ruth Bolletino and Dr Larry Leshan offer psychotherapy via Skype for international clients – www.cancerasaturningpoint.org.

17. Hamilton, D. R., *How Your Mind Can Heal Your Body*, Hay House, 2010 (p. 71).

Chapter 4

1. Spreen, A., *Tomorrow's Cancer Cures Today*, Health Sciences Institute, 2009 (p. 133).

2. http://www.ncbi.nlm.nih.gov/pubmed/1962588.

3. Murata, A. and Morishige, F., International Conference on Nutrition, Taijin, China 1981. Report in *Medical Tribune*, 22 June 1981, *International Journal for Vitamin and Nutrition Research*, 1982, A. Murata, et al., 'Prolongation of survival times of terminal cancer patients by administration of large doses of ascorbate', *International Journal for Vitamin and Nutrition Research*, supplement, 1982, 23, pp. 103–13.

4. www.ncbi.nlm.nih.gov/pubmed/20570889; www.nzherald.co.nz/nz/news/article.cfm?c_id=1&objectid=10659956.

5. www.aacr.org/home/about-us.aspx.

6. PMID:7366735 (and in particular, *Nature*, 17 April 1980, 284(5757), pp. 629–31, 'Vitamin C preferential toxicity for malignant melanoma cells').

7. Kang, J. S., Cho, D., Kim, Y. I., Hahm, E., Kim, Y. S., Jin, S. N., Kim, H. N., Kim, D., Hur, D., Park, H., Hwang, Y. I., Lee, W. J. J., 'Sodium ascorbate (vitamin C) induces apoptosis in melanoma cells via the down-regulation of transferrin receptor dependent iron uptake', *Journal of Cellular Physiology*, July 2005, 204(1), pp. 192–7.

8. www.townsendletter.com/Oct2004/warcancer1004.htm.

9. www.huffingtonpost.com/dr-mark-hyman/why-you-should-not-stop-t_b_1018430.html.

10. www.ncbi.nlm.nih.gov/pubmed/19054627.

11. mercola.fileburst.com/PDF/703-highly_cited_vitamin_D_cancer%5B3%5D.pdf.

12. articles.mercola.com/sites/articles/archive/2009/10/13/vitamin-d-doubles-colon-cancer-survival-rates.aspx.

13. Lappe, J. M., Travers-Gustafson, D., Davies, K. M., Recker, R. R., Heaney, R. P., 'Vitamin D and calcium supplementation reduces cancer risk: results of a randomized trial', *American Journal of Clinical Nutrition*, 2007, 85(6), pp. 1586–91.

14. articles.mercola.com/sites/articles/archive/2004/03/31/cancer-sunlight.aspx.

15. The Health Sciences Institute, 29 August 2012.

16. *Journal of Clinical Endocrinology & Metabolism*, 2010, www.nutra ingredients.com/Health-condition-categories/Cognitive-and-mental-function/Vitamin-D3-87-percent-more-potent-than-D2-Study.

17. www.drweil.com/drw/u/ART02812/vitamin-d.

18. www.globalhealingcenter.com/natural-health/10-foods-containing-vitamin-d/.

19. Brighthope, I., 'The Forces Against Health in Australia', *Orthomolecular Medicine News Service*, 25 June 2012, p 1.

20. gordonresearch.com/articles_vitamin_c/MNT_High_intravenous_vitamin_C_dose_fights_cancer.pdf.

21. Padayatty, S. J., Sun, H., Wang, Y., Riordan, H. D., Hewitt, S. M., Katz, A., Wesley, R. A., Levine, M., 'Vitamin C pharmacokinetics: implications for oral and intravenous use', *Annals of Internal Medicine*, 2004, 140, pp. 533–7; see also www.townsendletter.com/Oct2004/warcancer1004.htm.

22. www.doctoryourself.com/klennerbio.html.

23. www.3news.co.nz/Living-Proof-Vitamin-C—-Miracle-Cure/tabid/371/articleID/171328/Default.aspx.

24. http://informahealthcare.com/doi/abs/10.1080/135908408023 05423, Hickey, S., *Journal of Nutritional and Environmental Medicine*, 2008, 17(3), pp. 169–77 (doi:10.1080/13590840802305423).
25. http://ict.sagepub.com/content/7/4/223.extract.
26. Euler, L., *The Missing Ingredient for Good Health*, Online Publishing and Marketing, LLC 2007 (p. 9).
27. Ibid.
28. Ibid, p. 9.
29. ict.sagepub.com/content/7/4/223.full.pdf+html.
30. http://www.townsendletter.com/Oct2004/warcancer1004.htm.
31. See study from scientists from the US National Institutes of Health: Padayatty, S. J., Sun, H., Wang, Y., Riordan, H. D., Hewitt, S. M., Katz, A., Wesley, R. A., Levine, M., 'Vitamin C pharmacokinetics: implications for oral and intravenous use', *Annals of Internal Medicine*, 2004, 140, pp. 533–7.
32. Davies, S., 'Nutritional Flat-earthers', *Journal of Nutritional and Environmental Medicine*, 1990, 1:3, pp. 167–70.

Chapter 5

1. Interview with Gonzalez.
2. *Nutrition and Cancer*, 1999, 33(2), pp. 117–24; PMID: 10368805 (www.dr-gonzalez.com/pilot_study_abstract.htm).
3. Other experts like Dr Robert Jay Rowen claim the cure rate was 30–35 per cent.
4. www.ncbi.nlm.nih.gov/pubmed/9359807.
5. www.sciencedirect.com/science/article/pii/S0304383596044618.
6. www.ncbi.nlm.nih.gov/pubmed/3136944.
7. drhyman.com/blog/conditions/glutathione-the-mother-of-all-antioxidants/
8. Chris Kresser.
9. Patrick Holford.
10. drhyman.com/blog/conditions/glutathione-the-mother-of-all-anti oxidants/.
11. Ibid.
12. www.lifewave.com/pdf/Research/Research-HumanClinicalPilot Study.pdf.
13. Complementary and Alternative Medicine.
14. www.coffee-enema.ca/eforenema.htm.
15. www.dailymail.co.uk/femail/article-2275667/We-live-coffee-enemas-Meet-couple-inject-caffeine-colons-times-DAY.html.
16. www.huffingtonpost.co.uk/2012/04/18/simon-cowell-enemas_n_1433432.html.

17. Lechner, P. and Kronberger, L., 'Experiences with the use of dietary therapy in surgical oncology', *Aktuelle Ernaehrungsmedizin*, 1990, 2(15).

Chapter 6

1. Hyman, M., *The Blood Sugar Solution*, Hodder & Stoughton, 2012 (p. 247).
2. According to Dr Mark Hyman most of the 80,000 plus new chemicals and toxins on the market since 1900 have never been proven safe: Hyman, M., *The Blood Sugar Solution*, Hodder & Stoughton, 2012 (p. 247).
3. www.manchester.ac.uk/aboutus/news/display/?id=6243.
4. Kolata, G., 'New Ability to Find Earliest Cancers: A Mixed Blessing?' *New York Times*, 8 November 1994, www.nytimes.com/1994/11/08/ science/new-ability-to-find-earliest-cancers-a-mixed-blessing.html? pagewanted=all&src=pm.
5. Had the tumours been picked up while the woman was alive, they would have been labelled as breast cancer.
6. Reuben, Suzanne H., 'Reducing Environmental Cancer Risk: What We Can Do Now', for the President's Cancer Panel, April 2010 (deainfo.nci.nih.gov/advisory/pcp/annualReports/pcp08-09rpt/PCP_Report_08-09_508.pdf).
7. Buttar, R. A., *The 9 Steps to Keep the Doctor Away*, GMEC, 2010.
8. Malkan, S., *Not Just a Pretty Face: The Ugly Side of the Beauty Industry*, New Society Publishers, 2007 (p. 2).
9. See Clair Patterson, California Institute of Technology: www.caltech. edu/content/scientific-pioneer-clair-c-patterson-dies.
10. Lustberg, M., Silbergeld, E., 'Blood Lead Levels and Mortality' *Archives of Internal Medicine*, November 2002, 162(21) (archinte.jamanetwork.com/article.aspx?articleid=214370).
11. Rogers, S. A., *Detoxify or Die*, Prestige Publishing, 2002.
12. Douglass, W. C., *The Douglass Report*, August 2012, 12(4).
13. Hubbard, S., 'BPA: The Poison the Government Allows in Your Food', *Health Radar*, June 2012, 2(6), p. 6.
14. Link found between BPA and meningioma – a type of brain tumour. Douglass, W. C., *The Douglass Report*, October 2012, 12(6).
15. 'Radiation exposure from CT scans in childhood and subsequent risk of leukaemia and brain tumours: a retrospective cohort study', *Lancet*, Early Online Publication, 7 June 2012, doi:10.1016/S0140-6736(12)60815-0.
16. Buttar, R. A., *The 9 Steps to Keep the Doctor Away*, GMEC, 2010 (p. 260).
17. Ibid, p. 25.

18. www.epa.gov/oswer/vaporintrusion/documents/oswer-vapor-intrusion-background-Report-062411.pdf.

19. People Against Cancer provides up-to-date information for people about how to protect themselves from poisons in their food, air, water and environment.

20. A report released in 2008 from the Maine Department of Environmental Protection revealed that when a CFL bulb is broken, it can release dangerously high levels of mercury into the air: www.naturalnews.com/028034_mercury_compact_fluorescent_lights.html.

21. www.annieappleseedproject.org/drurjaalpakl.html.

22. Adams, P. J. D., '19 Ways Cancer Becomes the Ultimate Soft-Kill Operation', *Activist Post*, 17 July 2012, www.activistpost.com/2012/07/19-ways-cancer-becomes-ultimate-soft.html.

23. Douglass, W. C., *The Douglass Report*, August 2012, 12(4).

24. Chunyang Liao, Fang Liu and Kurunthachalam Kannan, *Environmental Science & Technology*, 2012, 46 (12), pp. 6515–22. http://portal.acs.org/portal/acs/corg/content?_nfpb=true&_page Label=PP_ARTICLEMAIN&node_id=223&content_id=CNBP_03026 4&use _sec=true&sec_url_var=region1&__uuid=32bb111c-bfc3-4f38-a403- 76c5c8c02d2d.

25. Press release, Natural Resources Defense Council, 'New study: Common air fresheners contain chemicals that may affect human reproductive development', September 2007, www.nrdc.org/media/2007/070919.asp; press release, News Target, 'Consumer alert: Popular air fresheners found to contain toxic chemical', 2007, www.newstarget.com.

26. Douglass, W. C., *The Douglass Report*, August 2012, 12(4).

27. News Release, Swedish Research Council, May 2012 (consumer.healthday.com/Article.asp?AID=665061).

28. Yeomans, M., 'Denmark bans four phthalates despite EU decision', August 2012, www.cosmeticsdesign-europe.com/Regulation-Safety/Denmark-bans-four-phthalates-despite-EU-decision/.

29. MacDonald, E., 'Formaldehyde classified as a carcinogen by HHS', *Consumer News*, June 2011, news.consumerreports.org/safety/2011/06/formaldehyde-classified-as-a-carcinogen-by-hhs.html.

30. Available from www.healthy-house.co.uk.

31. Carpenter, S., 'Want to reduce BPA exposure? Cut canned foods from your diet, report says', *Los Angeles Times*, March 2011 (latimesblogs.latimes.com/greenspace/2011/03/bpa-canned-food.html).

32. Douglass, W. C., *The Douglass Report*, August 2012, 12(4).

33. Grace, J. L., *Look Great Naturally . . . Without Ditching the Lipstick*, Hay House, 2012 (p. 248).
34. Harter Pierce, T., *Outsmart your cancer*, Thoughtworks Publishing, 2009 (p. 28).
35. 'Perchlorate, also known as the "rocket fuel chemical" . . . is frequently found contaminating the water supply', Adams, M., 'Banned toxic chemicals found in 100 per cent of pregnant women – new study', *Natural News*, January 2011, http://www.natural news.com/031033_toxic_chemicals_pregnant_women.html.
36. De Roos, A. J., Blair, A., Rusiecki, J. A., Hoppin, J. A., Svec, M., Dosemeci, M., Sandler, D. P., Alavanja, M. C., 'Cancer incidence among glyphosate-exposed pesticide applicators in the Agricultural Health Study', *Environmental Health Perspective*, January 2005, www.ncbi.nlm.nih.gov/pubmed/15626647.
37. Antoniou, M., et al., 'Teratogenic Effects of Glyphosate-Based Herbicides: Divergence of Regulatory Decisions from Scientific Evidence', *Journal of Environmental and Analytical Toxicology*, 2012, S4:006. doi:10.4172/2161-0525.S4-006.
38. Huff, E. A., 'Study: Roundup diluted by 99.8 per cent still destroys human DNA', *Natural News*, February 2012, www.naturalnews.com/035050_Roundup_Monsanto_DNA.html.
39. Ibid.
40. Tao, X. G., et al., 'Effects of drinking water from the lower reaches of the Huangpu River on the risk of male stomach and liver cancer death', Public Health Rev. 1991–2, 19 (1–4), pp. 229–36, www.ncbi.nlm.nih.gov/pubmed/1844271.
41. Group, E., 'Chlorine, Cancer, And Heart Disease', Global Healing Centre (www.globalhealingcenter.com/health-hazards-to-know-about/chlorine-cancer-and-heart-disease).
42. Ibid.
43. For many years France has used ozone to purify its water www.santelife.com/our-products/ozone-purification-systems/why-ozone/.
44. Altman, N., *The Oxygen Prescription: The Miracle of Oxidative Therapies*, Healing Arts Press, 2007.
45. Group, E., 'Chlorine, Cancer, And Heart Disease', Global Healing Centre (www.globalhealingcenter.com/health-hazards-to-know-about/chlorine-cancer-and-heart-disease).
46. According to research from the University of Western Australia (www.apostle.com.au/mediaarticles/).
47. Mercola, J., 'How Drinking More Spring or Filtered Water Can Improve Every Facet of Your Health', www.mercola.com/article/water.htm.

48. www.marksandspencer.com/Food-Manufacturing-Our-Food-Policies-About-Our-Food-MS-Foodhall-Food-Wine/b/46528031.
49. www.legislation.gov.uk/uksi/1990/2489/made.
50. www.bbc.co.uk/news/science-environment-20540758.
51. Harlander, S., 'Safety Assessments and Public Concern for Genetic-ally Modified Food Products: The American View', *Toxicologic Pathology*, 2002, 30(1), pp. 132–4.
52. 'How Some People Live to the Age of 100, 122, or Even 150 Years Old', *Underground Health Reporter*, newsletter, 22 October 2012, Think-Outside-the-Book Publishing, LLC.
53. Amos, J., 'French GM-fed rat study triggers furore', BBC News, 19 September 2012, (www.bbc.co.uk/news/science-environment-19654825).
54. www.foodmatters.tv/articles-1/gm-corn-linked-to-cancer-tumors.
55. Schubert, J., Riley, E. J., Tyler, S. A., 'Combined effects in toxicology. A rapid systematic testing procedure: cadmium, mercury, and lead', *Journal of Toxicology and Environ Health*, 1978, 4(5/6), pp. 763–76.
56. Poulter, S., 'Cornflakes cancer scare: Cereal makers drop recycled cardboard boxes containing deadly oils', *Daily Mail*, 9 March 2011, www.dailymail.co.uk/health/article-1364068/Recycled-cereal-boxes-contain-dangerous-levels-cancer-causing-mineral-oils.html.
57. Douglass, W. C., 'All natural? More like all garbage! The stomach-churning truth about what's hiding in your food', *The Douglass Report*, July 2012, 12(3).
58. Issels, J., *Cancer: A Second Opinion: A Look at Understanding Controlling, and Curing Cancer*, Square One Publishers, 2005 (p. 122). Fact confirmed by Will Revak, co-founder of the Healthy Mouth World Summit (www.HealThyMouthSummit.com).
59. www.paracelsus.ch/.
60. www.rooted.tv/ReferencesRooted.html.
61. Ibid.
62. Sundqvist, in 1976, isolated eighty-eight species of bacteria from thirty-two root canals with periapical disease. Wu, M. K., Moorer, W. R., Wesselink, P. R., 'Capacity of anaerobic bacteria enclosed in a simulated root canal to induce inflammation', *International Endodontic Journal*, 1989, 22, pp. 269–77.
63. www.whale.to/d/root2.html.
64. amcofh.org/blog/dr-hal-huggins-receives-lifetime-achievement-award.
65. Chong, B. S., Pitt Ford, T. R., Watson, T. F., Wilson, R. F., 'Sealing ability of potential retrograde root filling materials', *Endodontics and Dental Traumatology*, December 1995, 11(6), pp. 264–9; Adamo, H. L., Buruiana, R., Schertzer, L., Boylan, R. J., 'A comparison of

MTA, Super-EBA, composite and amalgam as root-end filling materials using a bacterial microleakage model', *International Endodontic Journal*, May 1999, 32(3), pp. 197–203; Higa, R. K., Torabinejad, M., McKendry, D. J., McMillan, P. J., 'The effect of storage time on the degree of dye leakage of root-end filling materials', *International Endodontic Journal*, September 1994, 27(5), pp. 252–6; Peters, L. B., Harrison, J. W., 'A comparison of leakage of filling materials in demineralized and non-demineralized resected root ends under vacuum and non-vacuum conditions', *International Endodontic Journal*, November 1992, 25(6), pp. 273–8.

66. articles.mercola.com/sites/articles/archive/2013/02/05/mercury-un-treaty-abolishes-amalgam.aspx.

67. *Indian Journal of Dental Research*, January–March 2009, 20(1), pp. 47–51. PMID: 19336860.

68. Smith-Bindman, R., et al., 'Radiation dose associated with common computed tomography examinations and the associated lifetime attributable risk of cancer', *Archives of Internal Medicine*, 14 December 2009, 169(22), pp. 2078–86.

69. Faloon, W., 'Lethal Danger of CT Scans', *Life Extension Magazine*, August 2010 (www.lef.org/magazine/mag2010/aug2010_Lethal-Danger-of-CT-Scans_01.htm).

70. www.hsionline.com.

71. Lehman, C. D., et al., 'MRI evaluation of the contralateral breast in women with recently diagnosed breast cancer', *New England Journal of Medicine*, 29 March 2007, 356(13), pp. 1295–303; epub 28 March 2007.

72. Graham, Georgia, 'Phone urge hits every 6 minutes', *The Sunday Times*, 10 February 2013, www.thesundaytimes.co.uk/sto/news/uk_news/Tech/article1211247.ece.

73. www.canceriscurablenow.tv/newsletter/no-emf-far-inrared-sauna-new-breakthrough.

74. Buttar, R. A., *The 9 Steps to Keep the Doctor Away*, GMEC, 2010 (p. 270).

75. Davidson, J. A. [letter], *Medical Journal of Australia*, 5 January 1998; also p. 163 of Holford, P., *Say No to Cancer*, Piatkus, 2010.

76. Levis, A. G., Minicuci, N., Ricci, P., Gennaro, V., Garbisa, S., 'Mobile phones and head tumours. The discrepancies in cause-effect relationships in the epidemiological studies – how do they arise?' *Environmental Health*, 17 June 2011 (www.ncbi.nlm.nih.gov/pubmed/21679472).

77. Yang, L., Hao, D., Wang, M., Zeng, Y., Wu, S., Zeng, Y., 'Cellular Neoplastic Transformation Induced by 916 MHz Microwave Radiation', *Cellular and Molecular Neurobiology*, 7 March 2012; epub PMID: 22395787 (www.ncbi.nlm.nih.gov/pubmed/22395787).

78. International Agency for Research on Cancer and World Health Organization press release no. 208, 31 May 2011 (www.iarc.fr/en/media-centre/pr/2011/pdfs/pr208_E.pdf).

79. www.naturalrussia.com/pdfs/Carcinogen_list.pdf.

80. According to the National Cancer Institute.

81. www.ncbi.nlm.nih.gov/pubmed/20447989. A 2008 report released by the Working Group of the International Agency for Research on Cancer (IARC) concluded that some of the chemicals these workers are exposed to are 'probably carcinogenic to humans'.

82. www.cancer.gov/cancertopics/factsheet/Risk/hair-dyes#r2.

83. Malkan, S., *Not Just a Pretty Face: The Ugly Side of the Beauty Industry*, New Society Publishers, 2007 (p. 70).

84. Ibid p. 56.

85. Ibid p. 10.

86. Products used in the eye area, such as mascara, eyeliner and eyeshadows are allowed to have mercury-based preservatives in them (www.forresthealth.com/ImagesX/melisa.pdf=).

87. *Nature & Health* magazine, August–September 2012, p. 17.

88. safecosmetics.org/downloads/FemCare_fs_022411.pdf.

89. Parker-Pope, T., 'When Hormone Creams Expose Others to Risks', *New York Times*, 25 October 2010 (well.blogs.nytimes.com/2010/10/ 25/when-hormone-creams-expose-others-to-risks/).

90. Based on 2005 update, 59.7 per cent of personal care products analysed in the database contained estrogenic chemicals and other endocrine disruptors, 'Summary of Major Findings', *Skin Deep* (online), (cited 4 May, 2007).

91. Duncan, D. E., 'Science and Space', *National Geographic*, October 2006 (science.nationalgeographic.com/science/article/toxic-people.html).

92. http://www.dailymail.co.uk/news/article-513209/Toxic-airlines-Is-plane-trip-poisoning-you.html#ixzz2TB7eV0EA.

93. cancerdefeated.com/newsletters/The-TSA-and-Your-Health.html

94. www.foodmatters.tv/articles-1/walking-barefoot-might-be-an-essential-element-of-good-health: reported in the *Journal of Environmental and Public Health*: 'It is an established fact that the Earth's surface possesses a limitless and continuously renewed supply of free or mobile electrons ... Mounting evidence suggests that the Earth's negative potential can create a stable internal bioelectrical environment for the normal functioning of all body systems.'

95. cancerdefeated.com/newsletters/The-TSA-and-Your-Health.html.

96. easyhealthoptions.com/alternative-medicine/nutrition/seaweed-detox-protection-and-super-source-of-nutrients/.

97. Dr Chiu Nan Lai of the University of Texas Health Sciences Center in Houston presented a paper at the 1979 meeting of the American Chemical Society suggesting that wheatgrass has anti-cancer properties. Research showed that wheatgrass extracts decrease the ability of mutagens to cause cancer by as much as 99 per cent. Later studies showed that wheatgrass extract inhibited the cancer-causing effects of benzopyrene and methylcholanthrene: Scheer, *'Green Foods,' Better Nutrition for Today's Living 55* (1993): 46; Seibold, R. L., *Cereal Grass: What's in It for You*, Wilderness Community Foundation, 1990. Annotations from p. 217 of *Meals That Heal: A Nutraceutical Approach to Diet and Health* by Lisa Turner.

98. *Journal of Ethnopharmacology*, October 2001, 77(2–3), pp. 203–8; PMID: 11535365.

99. http://www.naturalnews.com/015232_zeolite_zeolites.htm l#ixzz271Tt8bgw.

100. Platt, D., Raz, A., 'Modulation of the lung colonization of B16-F1 melanoma cells by citrus pectin', *Journal of the National Cancer Institute*, 18 March 1992 (www.ncbi.nlm.nih.gov/pubmed/ 1538421).

Chapter 7

1. Hyman, M., *The Blood Sugar Solution*, Hodder & Stoughton, 2012 (p. 270); and in a 2005 clinical study by the University of Missouri, Kansas City, Sunlighten's Solocarbon heaters were shown to lower blood pressure through a programme of thirty-minute infrared sauna sessions three times per week, www.sunlighten.com/ blood_pressure.html. See also *Journal of the American Medical Association,* August 1981.

2. www.sunlighten.com/cell_health.html.

3. Lieberman, S., 'A Review of Whole Body Hyperthermia and the Experience of Klinik St. Georg,' *Townsend Letter*, August–September 2009 (www.klinik-st-georg.de/fileadmin/publikationen/en/a_ review_of_whole_body_hyperthermia_and_the_experience_of_ klinik-st-georg.pdf).

4. www.sunlighten.com/weight-loss.html.

5. Selvendiran, K., Kuppusamy, M. L., Ahmed, S., Bratasz, A., Meenakshisundaram, G., Rivera, B. K., Khan, M.,'Oxygenation inhibits ovarian tumor growth by downregulating STAT3 and cyclin-D1 expressions', *Cancer Biology & Therapy*, 15 August 2010, 10(4), pp. 386–90; http://www.ncbi.nlm.nih.gov/pubmed/ 20562529.

6. One study published in the journal *Cancer Research* in 2011 revealed that brisk walking halted the progress of early-stage prostate cancer. Another study, this time from a Harvard professor,

found that women who walked one to three hours a week at a moderate pace had a 20 per cent reduced risk of breast cancer death. For those who walked three to five hours a week, the risk was reduced by 50 per cent.

7. www.experiencefestival.com/wp/article/rebounding-for-the-elderly.

8. Cecchini, M., LoPresti, V., 'Drug residues stored in the body following cessation of use: impacts on neuroendocrine balance and behavior – use of the Hubbard sauna regimen to remove toxins and restore health', *Medical Hypotheses*, 2007, 68(4), pp. 868–79.

9. www.sunlighten.com/detox.html.

10. War veterans who'd been exposed to Agent Orange experienced improvement of symptoms such as joint pain following far infrared saunas (Roehm, 1983). See also Rogers, S. A., *Detoxify or Die*, Prestige Publishing, 2002 (p. 196).

11. According to Dr Ursula Jacob, www.annieappleseedproject.org/drurjaalpakl.html.

12. Sunlight therapies now offer a drug-free programme (and products) which claim to kill off blood-borne viruses while strengthening the immune system.

13. (*Circulation, 1995*) Via Rogers, S. A., *Detoxify or Die*, Prestige Pubishing, 2002 (p. 225).

14. Rogers, S. A., *Detoxify or Die*, Prestige Publishing, 2002 (p. 227).

15. A clinically tested brand of saunas.

16. Unsure where your sauna falls on the EMF spectrum? Freudenmann encourages you to buy a trifield meter, a device that measures EMF levels.

17. In 1918 G. L. Rohdenburg published a collection of potential spontaneous remission cases. Among the 302 cases, the majority of the spontaneous remissions occurred either after a surgery to partially de-bulk a malignant tumour or after an acute fever. Rohdenburg, G. L., 'Fluctuations in the growth of malignant tumors in man, with especial reference to spontaneous regression', *Journal of Cancer Research*, 1918, 3, pp. 192–221.

18. www.dailymail.co.uk/health/article-1313773/Can-fever-cure-cancer-Jordan-baffled-doctors-leukaemia-vanished-new-evidence-suggests-remarkable-explanation-.html.

19. www.cancer.gov/cancertopics/factsheet/Therapy/hyperthermia#r2.

20. www.clinicaltrials.gov/ct2/show/NCT00911079?term=hyperthermia&rank=2.

21. The study involved a type of hyperthermia called regional hyperthermia.

22. Scott-Mumby, K., *Cancer Research Secrets*, Scott-Mumby Wellness, 2010 (pp. 141–2).

23. Hospital referred to as *Fachklinik Dr. Herzog* in Germany.

24. Interview with Dr Herzog.
25. www.niim.com.au/sites/default/files/newsitems/melbobserver_ht_article.pdf.

Chapter 8

1. http://globocan.iarc.fr/factsheets/cancers/breast.asp#INCIDENCE.
2. bodyecology.com/articles/the-top-3-most-addicting-foods-why-they're-destroying-your-health-and-how-to-get-your-kids-off-them#.UH1Iu18M9E.
3. Larsson, S. C., Bergkvist, L., Wolk, A., 'Milk and lactose intakes and ovarian cancer risk in the Swedish Mammography Cohort', *American Journal of Clinical Nutrition*, 2004, 80, pp. 1353–7.
4. Faber, M. T., Jensen, A., Søgaard, M., et al., 'Use of dairy products, lactose, and calcium and risk of ovarian cancer – results from a Danish case-control study', *Acta Oncologica*, 2012, 51, pp. 454–64.
5. www.ncbi.nlm.nih.gov/pmc/articles/PMC1317071/.
6. In a study of colorectal cancer patients published in the November 2010 issue of the journal *Hepatogastroenterology*, those who consumed probiotics showed significantly higher natural-killer cell activity.
7. http://www.ncbi.nlm.nih.gov/pubmed/15749636.
8. http://www.ncbi.nlm.nih.gov/pubmed/19199784 and http://www.ncbi.nlm.nih.gov/pubmed/20405842.
9. http://www.ncbi.nlm.nih.gov/pubmed/18540113.
10. Taken verbatim from Holford's report. Stanford, J. L. et al., 'Prostate cancer trends 1973–1995', SEER Program, National Cancer Institute. NIH Pub. No. 99–4543. Bethesda, MD, 1999.
11. Van der Pols, J. C. et al., 'Childhood dairy intake and adult cancer risk: 65-y follow-up of the Boyd Orr cohort', *American Journal of Clinical Nutrition*, December 2007, 86(6), pp. 1722–9.
12. Young, N. J., Metcalfe, C., Gunnell, D., et al., 'A cross-sectional analysis of the association between diet and insulin-like growth factor (IGF)-I, IGF-II, IGF-binding protein (IGFBP)-2, and IGFBP-3 in men in the United Kingdom', *Cancer Causes & Control*, 2012, 6, pp. 907–17. Gonzalez, C. A., Riboli, E., 'Diet and cancer prevention: Contributions from the European Prospective Investigation into Cancer and Nutrition (EPIC) study', *European Journal of Cancer*, 2010, 46, pp. 2555–62.
13. Moschos, S. J., Mantzoros, C. S., 'The role of the IGF system in cancer: from basic to clinical studies and clinical applications', *Oncology*, 2002, 63(4), pp. 317–32.
14. Rincon, M., Rudin, E., Barzilai, N., 'The insulin/IGF-1 signaling in mammals and its relevance to human longevity', *Experimental Gerontology*, November 2005, 40(11), pp. 873–7.

15. Feskanich, D., Willett, W. C., Colditz, G. A., 'Calcium, vitamin D, milk consumption, and hip fractures: a prospective study among postmenopausal women', *American Journal of Clinical Nutrition*, 2003, 77, pp. 504–11.

16. Sonneville, K. R., Gordon, C. M., Kocher, M. S., Pierce, L. M., Ramappa, A., Field, A. E., 'Vitamin D, Calcium, and Dairy Intakes and Stress Fractures Among Female Adolescents', *Archives of Pediatrics & Adolescent Medicine*, published ahead of print, 5 March 2012.

17. institutefornaturalhealing.com/2011/09/milk-does-a-body-more-harm-than-good/.

18. http://www.naturalnews.com/039244_milk_aspartame_FDA_petition.html#ixzz2Lzp9bvti19. chriskresser.com.

20. http://douglassreport.com/2009/12/25/raw-milk/.

21. douglassreport.com/2008/02/13/bacteria-contaminated-milk-kills-3-people/; douglassreport.com/2012/03/21/cdc-uses-made-up-math-to-incite-raw-milk/.

22. http://www.naturalnews.com/035489_got_milk_celebrities_pus.html#ixzz28j55U1F2.

23. Daniel, Kaayla T., *The Whole Soy Story: The Dark Side of America's Favorite Health Food*, New Trends, 2005 (pp. 311–30).

24. http://blog.wholesoystory.com/2005/07/24/israeli-health-ministry-issues-soy-warning/.

25. Ji, Sayer, 'Are Cancer Stem Cells the Key to Discovering a Cure?' 8 May 2012, Green Med Info (www.greenmedinfo.com/blog/are-cancer-stem-cells-key-discovering-cure).

26. Linhing, Li and Neaves, William B., *Cancer Research*, 1 May 2006, 66 (9).

27. McCarron, K. and Chorsky, R., 'Reduction of Angiogenesis and Cell Doubling: Invasive Ductal Carcinoma of the Mammary Gland After 16 Days of Fermented Soy', Haelan Research Foundation.

28. *Townsend Newsletter*, June 2007.

29. Based on macrophage phagacytosis, www.haelanhopelessnomore.com/uploads/Haelan_Understanding_Breast_Cancer_Treatments_Wainright_2004.pdf.

30. Gocan, Anca G., Bachg, Doris, Schindler, A. E. and Rohr, U. D., 'Managing immunity in resistant cancer patients correlates to survival: results and discussion of a pilot study' *Hormone Molecular Biology and Clinical Investigation*, 2011, 8(2), pp. 455–69; see also Klein, A., He, X., Roche, M., Malett, A., Duska, L., Supko, J. G., Seiden, M. V., 'Prolonged stabilization of platinum resistant ovarian cancer in a single patient consuming a fermented soy therapy', *Gynecologic Oncology*, 2006, 100, pp. 205–9.

31. Spreen, A., *Tomorrow's Cancer Cures TODAY*, Health Sciences Institute, 2009 (p. 140).

32. Rohr, U. D., Li, W. W., Ziqiang, H., Wainright, W. Schindler, A. E., 'The effect of fermented soy (FSWW08) on blood hematology and cachexia in cancer patients', *Hormone Molecular Biology and Clinical Investigation*, 2012.

33. www.haelanhopelessnomore.com/uploads/Haelan_Understanding_Breast_Cancer_Treatments_Wainright_2004.pdf.

34. November 2004 Townsend Letter, *Soy and Cancer Survivors: Dietary Supplementation with Fermented Soy Nutraceutical, Haelan 951 in Patients Who Survived Terminal Cancers*.

35. In the paper Fermented Soy Research Mechanisms of Action eliediab.info/Haelan/Doc016%20-%20Mechanisms%20Of%20Action.pdf

36. www.haelanhopelessnomore.com/uploads/Haelan_Understanding_Breast_Cancer_Treatments_Wainright_2004.pdf.

37. www.alsearsmd.com/dont-put-this-in-your-starbucks/

38. *Scientific American* August 2009, www.alsearsmd.com/frankenstein-lurking-in-your-pantry/.

39. www.alsearsmd.com/frankenstein-lurking-in-your-pantry/.

40. www.bbc.co.uk/news/science-environment-19654825.

41. January 2012 wrightnewsletter.com/2012/01/30/dairy-industry-attacks-on-alternatives/.

42. bodyecology.com/articles/the-top-3-most-addicting-foods-why-they're-destroying-your-health-and-how-to-get-your-kids-off-them.

43. Researchers have found that nearly 50 per cent of patients admitted to an ICU in a tertiary cancer hospital presented with an abnormally low level of magnesium: Deheinzelin, D., Negri1, E. M., Tucci, M. R., Salem1, M. Z. da Cruz1, V. M., Oliveira, R. M., Nishimoto I. N., Hoelz, C., 'Hypomagnesemia in critically ill cancer patients: a prospective study of predictive factors', *Brazilian Journal of Medical and Biological Research*, December 2000, 33(12), pp. 1443–8.

Chapter 9

1. Lecture given at the meeting of the Nobel-Laureates on 30 June 1966 at Lindau, Lake Constance, Germany: healingtools.tripod.com/primecause1.html/.

2. www.thephillipdemarscancerfund.com/oxygentherapy.htm.

3. Harter Pierce, T., *Outsmart Your Cancer*, Thoughtworks Publishing, 2010 (p. 324).

4. Since 1822, the United States Department of Commerce and the US Department of Agriculture have kept yearly records on sweetener sales, such as cane sugar, high-fructose corn syrup and

maple syrup (http://bodyecology.com/articles/the-top-3-most-addicting-foods-why-they're-destroying-your-health-and-how-to-get-your-kids-off-them#.UH7Bqe18M9E).

5. 'The extracellular (interstitial) pH (pHe) of solid tumours is significantly more acidic compared to normal tissues', www.ncbi.nlm. nih.gov/pubmed/10362108?dopt=Abstrac; I discuss the pH theory in greater depth in Chapter 13.

6. According to Dr. Dan Cullum: www.naturalhealthcenterok.com/therapy/ozone.shtml.

7. Altman, N. *The Oxygen Prescription: The Miracle of Oxidative Therapies*, Healing Arts Press, 2007.

8. Warrington, R. 'The LA cult of kale comes to Britain', *The Times*, 16 February 2013, www.thetimes.co.uk/tto/life/food/article3688699.ece.

9. Many famous buildings, sculptures and paintings have been designed according to the Golden Ratio.

10. www.experiencefestival.com/wp/article/rebounding-for-the-elderly.

11. You can find a list of Dr Rowen's trainees at www.doctorrowen.com.

12. www.oxygenhealingtherapies.com/ozone_oxygen_therapies.html.

13. www.naturalhealthcenterok.com/therapy/ozone.shtml.

14. According to Dr Francisco Contreras from the Oasis of Hope Clinic in Tijuana Mexico, www.oasisofhope.com/ozone-therapy.php.

15. www.revistaespañoladeozonoterapia.es/index.php/reo/article/view/24/24.

16. Ibid.

17. Diaz-Llera, S., González-Hernández, Y., Mesa, J. E. G., Martínez-Sánchez, G. Re, L., 'Induction of DNA primary damage in peripheral blood leukocytes and exfoliated colorectal epithelial cells in rats treated with O3/O2 mix', *International Journal of Ozone Therapy*, 2009, 8, pp. 217–21; Guanche, et al., 'Effect of ozone/oxygen mixture on systemic oxidative stress and organic damage', *Toxicology Mechanisms and Methods*, January 2010, 20(1), pp. 25–30.

18. www.ncbi.nlm.nih.gov/pubmed/15770045.

19. Euler, L. and Scholberg, A., 'The Healing Power of Light Known for 84 Years, Ignored by Mainstream Medicine', *Cancer Defeated!* newsletter 235 (cancerdefeated.com/newsletters/This-light-therapy-really-IS-a-miracle-cure.html).

20. Wright, J. V., 'Harnessing the Power of Light', *Nutrition & Healing*, vol. 15, issue 3, May 2008, p. 4 and Gaiseniuk, L. A., 'Use of re-infusions of isolated irradiated auto-blood for the correction of hematopoietic disorders', *Med Radiol* (Mosk), November 1987, 32(11), pp. 15–18.

21. Roguski, J. P., *The Truth about Food Grade Hydrogen Peroxide*, Under the Radar Publishing, 2009, www.FoodGrade-HydrogenPeroxide.com (p 4).

22. Collins, D. 'The World's Greatest Healing Miracle of All Time', 9 June 2012 via *Cancer Defeated!* newsletter.

23. www.1minutecure.com/videofullstory4toindexnooptin.htm.

24. Roguski, J. P., *The Truth about Food Grade Hydrogen Peroxide*, Under the Radar Publishing, 2009, www.FoodGrade-HydrogenPeroxide.com (p. 2).

25. M. C. Symonds, et al., 'Hydrogen Peroxide: A Potent Cytotoxic Agent Effective in 26 Causing Cellular Damage and Used in the Possible Treatment for Certain Tumors', *Medical Hypothesis*, July 2001, 57, pp. 56–8.

26. www.cancertutor.com/Cancer/HydrogenPeroxide.html.

Chapter 10

1. National Cancer Institute: Surveillance Epidemiology End Results (SEER) Cancer Statistics Review, http://seer.cancer.gov/statfacts/html/all.html.

2. www.patient.co.uk/doctor/carcinoembryonic-antigen-cea.

3. A study on biopsy risk in the *American Journal of Surgical Pathology* reported that 'Tumor cell displacement was observed in 32 per cent of patients who had undergone large-gauge needle core biopsy of the breast. Fine-needle aspiration may shed breast cells into peripheral blood.'

4. Berrington de González, A., Mahesh, M., Kim, K. P., et al., 'Projected cancer risks from computed tomographic scans performed in the United States in 2007', *Archives of Internal Medicine*, 14 December 2009, 169(22), pp. 2071–7; www.lef.org/magazine/ mag2010/aug2010_Lethal-Danger-of-CT-Scans_01.htm.

5. Heterocyclic amines.

6. In 2008 the most common cancer among males in most economically developed countries was prostate, with the exception of Japan where stomach cancer was the most common (Global Cancer Facts & Figures – American Cancer Society www.cancer.org/acs/groups/content/@epidemiologysurveilance/documents/document/acspc-027766.pdf).

7. www.ncepod.org.uk/2008report3/Downloads/SACT_report.pdf #search='chemotherapy; www.abc.net.au/news/2008-11-13/chemotherapy-contributes-to-a-quarter-of-cancer/204358.

8. Quoted by Dr Garry Gordon and Kobayashi (saihatsuyobou.com/lpen/).

9. *Journal of Oncology*, 2004, Via Forsythe, J. W., *Take Control of Your Cancer*, BenBella Books, 2012 (p. 114).

10. Goetz, T., 'Why Early Detection Is the Best Way to Beat Cancer', *Wired Magazine,* 22 December 2008, www.wired.com/medtech/ health/magazine/17-01/ff_cancer?currentPage=all.
11. According to the Canary Foundation, a non-profit organisation dedicated to early cancer detection.
12. A description a friend of mine shared, following a course of chemotherapy.
13. http://www.rational-t.com/patient-stories/default.aspx?id=13.
14. www.forresthealth.com/ImagesX/melisa.pdf.
15. Andraka won the $75,000 Gordon E. Moore award at the Intel International Science and Engineering Fair.

Chapter 11

1. http://www.youtube.com/watch?v=PZpRP1FV0lE.
2. Claude Swanson.
3. Dr Alex Loyd.
4. Master Li.
5. www.synchronizeduniverse.com/about_book.htm.
6. www.u-energy.org/ScienceTest/DistanceHealing2007.html.
7. Scott-Mumby, K., *Cancer Research Secrets*, Scott-Mumby Wellness, 2010 (p. 266).
8. Taken from an interview with Dr Claude Swanson: http://www.youtube.com/watch?v=ZVjtiJOGcPs.
9. Taken from essay 'Cancer a Redox Disease', *The Institute of Science in Society*, 2012, www.i-sis.org.uk/Cancer_a_Redox_Disease.php.
10. Studies show that many of us are deficient in this key mineral – including 80 per cent of Americans (Shealy, N., *Energy Medicine*, 4th Dimension Press, 2011 (p. 161).
11. Acupuncture: Review and Analysis of Reports on Controlled Clinical Trials, apps.who.int/medicinedocs/pdf/s4926e/s4926e.pdf.
12. Dyczynski, J., 'The effective initial screening and monitoring of successful acupuncture intervention using the new European Cardio Stress Imaging Technology', *Australian Journal of Acupuncture and Chinese Medicine*, 2012, 7(2).
13. I have changed certain details in this story to protect the woman's anonymity.
14. totallyalive.com.au/.
15. www.innervisionsworldwide.com.
16. www.thesacredtree.com.au.
17. www.terryoconnell.com.
18. Incidentally, it was Terry's very first session as a theta practitioner.
19. undergroundhealthreporter.com/music-for-health-dna-repair#axzz2G9pPV69h.

20. www.ted.com/talks/bill_doyle_treating_cancer_with_electric_
fields.html.
21. www.sciencedirect.com/science/article/pii/S0006291X06004256, 5
May 2006, 343, (2), pp. 351–60.
22. For the treatment of depression.
23. www.earthinginstitute.net/studies/grounding_body_2000.pdf.
24. www.earthinginstitute.net/studies/earthing_pulse_rate.pdf.
25. www.chinadaily.com.cn/life/2010-01/08/content_9286317.htm.
26. www.nytimes.com/2013/05/12/opinion/sunday/the-hidden-world-
of-soil-under-our-feet.html?pagewanted=all&_r=0.
27. 24 June 1996 issue of *TIME Magazine* via Shealy, N., *Energy
Medicine*, 4th Dimension Press, 2011 (p. 271).

Chapter 12

1. In 2012 neuroscientists at the University of Wisconsin found that
long-term practitioners – those who have engaged in more than
50,000 rounds of meditation – showed significant changes in their
brain function, although those with only three weeks of 20-minute
meditation session per day also demonstrated some change;
blogs.smithsonianmag.com/smartnews/2012/11/the-worlds-
happiest-man-is-a-tibetan-monk/.
2. Frenkel, M., Ari, S. L., Engebretson, J., Peterson, N., Maimon, Y.,
Cohen, L., Kacen, L., 'Activism among exceptional patients with
cancer', *Supportive Care in Cancer*, August 2011, 19(8), pp. 1125–32.

Chapter 13

1. The cost of the average chemotherapy regimen: $300,000 to
$1,000,000 according to Dr Mark Sircus.
2. www.thedailybeast.com/newsweek/2012/08/26/the-cancer-
breakthroughs -that-cost-too-much-and-do-too-little.html.
3. The overall contribution of curative and adjuvant cytotoxic
chemotherapy to five-year survival in adults was estimated to be
2.3 per cent in Australia and 2.1 per cent in the USA, according to
a US government site, www.ncbi.nlm.nih.gov/pubmed/15630849.
4. www.ncbi.nlm.nih.gov/pubmed/11275453.
5. http://www.youtube.com/watch?v=3AJiRnirxxU; www.youtube.
com/user/CherylShumanTheOnly.
6. www.reuters.com/article/2012/05/31/us-drugs-science-research-
idUSBRE84U0DX20120531.
7. www.economist.com/news/finance-and-economics/21571898-
fund-seeks-opportunity-weed-audacity-dope?fsrc=scn/tw/te/dope.

8. Doblin, R. E. and Kleiman, M. A., *Journal of Clinical Oncology*, July 1991, 9(7), pp. 1314–19, http://jco.ascopubs.org/content/9/7/1314.abstract.

9. Sircus, M., *Medical Marijuana*, IMVA, 2012 (p. 47).

10. American Association for Cancer Research, 17 April 2007, 'Marijuana Cuts Lung Cancer Tumor Growth In Half, Study Shows', www.sciencedaily.com/releases/2007/04/070417193338.htm.

11. Sircus, M., *Medical Marijuana*, IMVA, 2012 (p. 48) and americanmarijuana.org/pot.shrinks.tumors.html.

12. Sircus, M., *Medical Marijuana*, IMVA, 2012 (p. 49).

13. en.wikipedia.org/wiki/Glioma.

14. Foroughi, M., Hendson, G., Sargent, M. A., Steinbok, P., 'Spontaneous regression of septum pellucidum/forniceal pilocytic astrocytomas – possible role of Cannabis inhalation', *The Child's Nervous System*, April 2011, 27(4), pp. 671–9; doi: 10.1007/s00381-011-1410-4. Epub 2011 Feb 20. www.ncbi.nlm.nih.gov/pubmed/21336992.

15. phoenixtears.ca/articles/hemp-the-most-medicinal-plant-in-the-world-in-action/.

16. abcnews.go.com/Health/montana-father-medical-marijuana-cancer-stricken-toddler-son/story?id=13529490.

17. www.thecannacig.com/.

18. www.alternet.org/drugs/media-ignored-experts-shocking-findings-marijuana-helps-prevent-lung-cancer-now-its-med-school?page=0%2C0.

19. 'The extracellular (interstitial) pH (pHe) of solid tumours is significantly more acidic compared to normal tissues.' www.ncbi.nlm.nih.gov/pubmed/10362108?dopt=Abstrac.

20. Robey, I. F., et al., 'Bicarbonate increases tumor pH and inhibits spontaneous metastases', *Cancer Research*, 2009, 69, p. 2260.

21. www.oasisofhope.com/sodium-bicarbonate.php.

22. *British Journal of Cancer*, 2012, 106(7), pp. 1280–87 (people.maths.ox.ac.uk/maini/PKM%20publications/330.pdf).

23. http://www.townsendletter.com/Dec2009/warcancer1209.html.

24. Gupta, S. C., Sung, B., Kim, J. H., Prasad, S., Li, S., Aggarwal, B. B., 'Multitargeting by turmeric, the golden spice: From kitchen to clinic', *Molecular Nutrition & Food Research*, 2012, Aug, pp. 1–19.

25. Collins, D., *The Top 10 Natural Cancer Cures No One is Talking About*, Think-Outside-the-Book Publishing, LLC, p. 21; http://www.Top10CancerCures.com.

26. Ibid, p. 22.

27. *Molecular Nutrition & Food Research*, 2012, Aug, pp. 1–19.

28. Used either alone or in combination with other agents, Gupta, S.

C., Patchva, S. and Aggarwal, B. B., 'Therapeutic Roles of Curcumin: Lessons Learned from Clinical Trial' the *AAPS Journal*, 2012.

29. Purkayastha, S., Berliner, A., Fernando, S. S., Ranasinghe, B., Ray, I., Tariq, H. and Banerjee P., 'Curcumin Blocks Brain Tumor Formation', *Brain Research*, 10 February 2009, www.ncbi.nlm.nih. gov/pubmed/19368804.

30. http://www.menshealth.com/health/tumeric-curing-disease# ixzz2I3fmCKLf.

31. curcuminresearch.org/response.html.

32. Name changed.

33. Bollinger, T. M., *Cancer – Step Outside The Box*, 5th Edition (p. 260).

34. Holford, P., *Say No to Cancer*, Piatkus, 2010 (p. 158).

35. www.ncbi.nlm.nih.gov/pubmed/10075116.

36. According to Dr Nicholas Perricone, when applied topically Curcuminoids can: '. . . provide the skin with many benefits, including increased radiance, decreased pore size, and, with continued use, a reduction in fine lines and discolouration', *Nature & Health Magazine*, April–May 2012.

37. This list of chemotherapy agents was provided by Aggarwal.

38. Gray, L., 'Marchioness of Worcester: organic diet helped me beat breast cancer', the *Telegraph*, 30 December 2012, www.telegraph. co.uk/earth/earthnews/9771839/Marchioness-of-Worcester-organic-diet-helped-me-beat-breast-cancer.html.

39. Holford, P., *Say No to Cancer*, Piatkus, 2010 (p. 130).

40. http://undergroundhealthreporter.com/salvestrols-a-natural-anti-cancer-chemicals-found-in-every-day-fruits#ixzz2IF17tSef.

41. The *Telegraph* recently reported that these 800-year-old apples are the healthiest to eat, www.telegraph.co.uk/health/healthnews/6151010/800-year-old-apple-healthiest-to-eat.html.

42. Frenkel, M., Mishra, B. M., Sen, S., Yang, P., Pawlus, A., Vence, L., Leblanc, A., Cohen, L., Banerjee P. Banerji, P., *International Journal of Oncology*, February 2010, 36(2), pp. 395–403, www.ncbi.nlm.nih. gov/pubmed/20043074.

43. www.moshefrenkelmd.com/index.asp?page=2058&lang=eng.

44. Frenkel, M., Mishra, B. M., Sen, S., Yang, P., Pawlus, A., Vence, L., Leblanc, A., Cohen, L., Banerjee, P. and Banerji P. *International Journal of Oncology*, February 2010, 36(2), pp. 395–403, www.ncbi.nlm.nih.gov/pubmed/20043074.

45. Ibid.

46. Downer, S. M., et al., 'Pursuit and practice of complementary therapies by cancer patients receiving conventional treatment', *BMJ*, 1994, 309(6947), pp. 86–9.

47. Träger-Maury, S., et al., 'Use of complementary medicine by cancer patients in a French oncology department' [article in French], *Bulletin du Cancer*, 2007, 94(11), pp. 1017–25.
48. Johannessen, H., von Bornemann Hjelmborg, J., Pasquarelli, E., Fiorentini, G., Di Costanzos, F., Miccinesi, G., 'Prevalence in the use of complementary medicine among cancer patients in Tuscany, Italy', *Tumori*, 2008, 94(3). pp. 406–10.
49. 'Ruta 6 selectively induces cell death in brain cancer cells but proliferation in normal peripheral blood lymphocytes: A novel treatment for human brain cancer', *International Journal of Oncology*, 2003, 23, pp. 975–82. www.ncbi.nlm.nih.gov/pubmed/12963976.
50. Hubbard, B. 'Much more than a placebo: Homeopathy reverses cancer' *WDDTY*, March 2012, 22 (12), pp. 10–14.
51. Frenkel, M., Ari, S. L., Engebretson, J., Peterson, N., Maimon, Y., Cohen, L., Kacen L., 'Activism among exceptional patients with cancer', *Supportive Care in Cancer*, August 2011,19(8), pp. 1125–32.

On Love and Loss

1. Siegel, B., *Peace, Love and Healing,* Rider, 1999.

Resources

Chapter 1: Accept the Diagnosis Not the Prognosis

Practitioners and advice

Laura Bond: Confused about food or feeling stuck in a rut? As a health coach, I will work with you, one to one, to help you achieve your goals – whether it's building a stronger immune system, kicking a sugar habit or getting on top of emotional stress. I have trained with the Institute for Integrative Nutrition – the largest nutrition school in the world. www.laura-bond.com.

To have Laura or Gemma Bond speak at your next event go to www.MumsNotHavingChemo.com.

Shannon Burford: at his clinic in Perth, Western Australia, Burford aims to educate, empower and support patients to obtain optimum health. He practises herbal and nutritional medicine and uses an extensive range of investigative tests. Consultations are available Australia-wide via Skype or telephone. www.naturalcancertreatments.com.au

Credence Publications: set up by health author Phillip Day, this independent research organisation is dedicated to reporting properly annotated and verified information to enable readers to make wise health decisions. www.credence.org

David Getoff: there is typically a five- to eight-week waiting list for private consultations with this health educator, clinical nutritionist and star of *Food Matters*. www.naturopath4you.com

Dr Garry Gordon: the website of this highly respected medical doctor provides cutting-edge research on energy medicine, enzymes, high-dose vitamin C, chelation, PEMF and more. You will also find an invaluable database of practitioners trained in environmental and nutritional medicine. www.gordonresearch.com

Dr Patrick Kingsley: Dr Kingsley is the author of over 30 books, most of which are on cancer, all of which are available on Amazon Kindle and his website, where you can learn how to overcome chronic disease without drugs or surgery. www.thenewmedicine.info

Ralph W. Moss, PhD: the acclaimed medical writer and researcher now offers phone consultations to help patients find an individualized approach to cancer treatment. www.cancerdecisions.com

Dr Mark Sircus: Dr Sircus offers one-on-one consultations and online support programmes through which you will have access to him and his staff on a daily basis. His website should also be the first port of call for those looking for natural, affordable treatment options. www.drsircus.com

What Doctors Don't Tell You (*WDDTY*): brainchild of best-selling author Lynne McTaggart and husband Bryan Hubbard, *WDDTY* magazine is an invaluable resource for anyone wanting to expand their knowledge of natural medicine. The website also offers a database of UK-based practitioners from a wide range of disciplines from colonic irrigation to bioenergetic testing. www.wddty.com

Chapters 2 and 3: The Cancer Personality and The Cancer Survivor

Emotional support

Thanks to the pioneering work of people like Bernie Siegel and Lawrence LeShan there are now cancer support groups available worldwide. I encourage you to find programmes, retreats and services in your local community that will help heal your body and nourish your spirit.

UK

Patrizia Sergeant is a UK-based healer who practises the Journey process, Bowen Technique, reiki and past-life therapy: www.patriziasergeant.co.uk/

Australia

Based in Perth, Casey Terry uses various healing modalities to transform belief patterns and release old, unwanted energies. She also runs healing and coaching sessions and workshop programmes across Australia and internationally: totallyalive.com.au

USA

Lawrence LeShan, Ruth Bolletino and Mary Bobis offer psychotherapy and counselling for people dealing with cancer, including family caregivers and former cancer patients, residential workshops throughout the USA, as well as telephone or Skype sessions for people abroad: www.cancerasaturningpoint.org

Worldwide

Dr Leonard Coldwell's Instinct Based Medicine System (IBMS™): Dr Coldwell is considered a leading authority in self-help education for cancer patients. His best-selling books, CDs and DVDs provide stress reduction through a combination of words and healing frequencies: www.instinctbasedmedicine.com

Books

Barasch, M. I., *The Healing Path* (Penguin, 1995)

Bays, B., *The Journey* (Harper Element, 2003)

Buttar, R. A., *The 9 Steps To Keep The Doctor Away* (GMEC, 2010)

Hay, L., *You Can Heal Your Life* (Hay House, 2004)

Marson, J., *The Curse of Lovely* (Piatkus, 2013)

Moore, T., *Dark Nights of the Soul* (Piatkus, 2011)

Moritz, A., *Cancer is Not a Disease: It's a Survival Mechanism* (Ener-chi.com, 2005)

Myss, C., *Anatomy of the Spirit* (Bantam Books, 1997)

Myss, C., *Self Esteem: Your Fundamental Power* (Sounds True, 2006)

Nelson, B., *The Emotion Code* (Wellness Unmasked Publishing, 2007)

Siegel, B., *Peace, Love & Healing* (Rider, 1999)

www.healingcancer.info/ebook/lawrence-leshan

(For more inspiring advice, look out for Dr Kelly Turner's new book *Radical Remission*.)

Chapter 4: Vitamin Injections

Treatment with or information about intravenous vitamin C

UK

Dr Wendy Denning: Dr Denning is a GP with over twenty-five years' experience. Passionate about the integration of traditional and complementary medicine and clued up on cutting-edge diagnostics, she will always offer a keen ear and big smile: www.thehealthdoctors.co.uk

Yes to Life: the charity provides a directory of physicians trained in complementary and alternative medicine including intravenous vitamin C, mistletoe and hyperthermia: www.yestolife.org.uk

The British Society for Ecological Medicine: physicians trained to take into account nutritional and environmental influences on health and chemical sensitivities: www.ecomed.org.uk

Australia and New Zealand

The Australasian College of Nutritional and Environmental Medicine: www.acnem.org

Note: Professor Brighthope is no longer consulting and cannot give medical advice to a patient not under his care.

USA

The Academy for Comprehensive Integrative Medicine:
www.acimconnect.com/

American Association of Naturopathic Physicians:
www.naturopathic.org

The International College of Integrative Medicine:
www.icimed.com

The American College for Advancement in Medicine:
www.acamnet.org

Worldwide

Orthomolecular.org: orthomolecular medicine aims to restore the
optimum environment of the body by addressing imbalances, using
natural substances such as vitamins, minerals and amino acids.

Vitamin C products

Bio En'R-G'y C and VitaChek-C urine test strips:
www.longevityplus.com

Lypo-spheric vitamin C: British readers can go to
www.lyposphericnutrients.co.uk and Australians can purchase the
product at www.livonlabs.com

Vitamin D

The dminder app for iPhone tracks the vitamin D you get from the
sun: www.dminder.info/

Real Sunlight: find 'natural sunlight' in various locations across the
UK whatever the weather: www.realsunlight.co.uk

Oral vitamin D3 spray: www.betteryou.uk.com

Books and DVDs

Food Matters: the groundbreaking documentary spills the beans
on the reality of the food industry and discusses a range of

natural treatments for chronic illness including intravenous vitamin C.

Collins, D., *The Top 10 Natural Cancer Cures* (Think-Outside-the-Book Publishing, Inc., 2011)

Euler, L., *The Missing Ingredient for Good Health* (Online Publishing and Marketing, 2007)

Holford, P., *Say No To Cancer* (Piatkus, 2010)

Kingsley, P., *The New Medicine* (Abaco Publishing, 2011)

Pitchford, P., *Healing with Whole Foods: Asian Traditions and Modern Nutrition* (North Atlantic Books, 2002)

Chapter 5: How Do You Take Your Coffee?

Expert support

Dr Nicholas Gonzalez: known as the coffee enema king, Dr Gonzalez regularly speaks at international conferences and his research has appeared in peer-reviewed medical journals: www.dr-gonzalez.com

Kathryn Alexander: Alexander conducts long-distance consultations from Australia about detoxification and Gerson Therapy: www.kathrynalexander.com.au

Quality coffee

UK

Buy 'Gerson blend' coffee online through Coffee Plant in London: www.coffee.uk.com

Worldwide

S. A. Wilsons sells organic gold roast coffee specially blended and roasted to have the highest levels of caffeine and palmitic acid available; free shipping to Canada, New Zealand and Australia: www.sawilsons.com

Enema equipment

www.enemaequipment.com

www.enemasupply.com/coltubin3siz.html

The Raw Food World: detox crusader Matt Monarch sells everything from juicers and chemical-free make-up to high-quality coconut oil and enema bags. Monarch has developed a worldwide following thanks to his informative, honest and always inspiring videos. www.therawfoodworld.com

See also www.Manifesthealth.co.uk

Cellgevity is available at www.masgxl.com

Books

Alexander, K., *Dietary Healing: the complete detox program* (Annexus Pty, Limited, 2013)

Alexander, K., *Nutritional Healing: a Patient Management Handbook* (Annexus Pty, Limited, 2013)

Gonzalez, N., *What Went Wrong: The Truth Behind the Clinical Trial of the Enzyme Treatment of Cancer* (New Spring Press, 2012)

Rogers, S. A., *Detoxify or Die* (Prestige Publishing, 2002)

For further tips and advice regarding coffee enemas visit the Gerson Institute's website (www.gerson.org); you will also find detailed information about the Gerson Therapy clinics in Mexico and Hungary.

Chapter 6: Getting Clean

In your home; in your water

UK

The Cancer Prevention and Education Society: www.cancerpreventionsociety.org

Choose Greeen: deals on organic restaurants, low carbon electrical products, soft furnishings and more: www.choosegreen.co.uk

Green Shop: specialises in eco-building products, consultation and services, natural paints, sustainable energy solutions, as well as organic and fairtrade bodycare and cleaning products: www.greenshop.co.uk/

Healthy House: earthing sheets, organic paints (including anti-formaldehyde radiator paint), pollution protection sprays, reverse osmosis filters and more: www.healthy-house.co.uk

Pureshowers: extensive range of chlorine and chemical-quashing filters: Pureshowers.co.uk

Australia

Ecolour Non Toxic Paint: with 36,000 colours available, this website offers NO VOCs paints delivered Australia-wide: www.ecocolour.com.au

Vitality4Life: for water filters, oxygen generators, air purifiers, kitchenware, infrared saunas, along with cold-pressed juicers, wheatgrass kits and more. International shipping available: www.vitality4life.co.uk and www.vitality4life.com.au/

USA

American Board of Clinical Metal Toxicology: www.abcmt.org

Delos Building Wellness: a company which creates healthy living and office spaces, with wellness guru Deepak Chopra on the advisory board: www.delosliving.com

Eco Choices Natural Living: everything from bamboo flooring to cast-iron cookware: www.ecochoices.com/

Gaiam: extensive range of natural homeware, along with consciousness-raising DVDs and yoga gear: www.gaiam.com

People Against Cancer: this grass-roots organisation provides the latest information on how to protect yourself from poisons in food, the air, water and environment: www.PeopleAgainstCancer.org

In your food

You can now find natural health-food stores on every corner in every major city in the world:

In London, Planet Organic is my favourite haunt. Opened in 1995, it is the UK's largest fully certified organic supermarket and now boasts three centrally located stores; you can also order online: www.planetorganic.com

In Perth, Western Australia, mum likes to stock up on fresh produce at Manna Wholefoods, www.mannawholefoods.com.au and Precious Organics: www.preciousorganics.com.au. Pure Health, run by naturopath Sharon Blackman, is also stacked with organic superfoods and high-quality supplements: www.purehealthclaremont.com.au

In the USA Wholefoods has almost single-handedly brought healthy eating to the masses. This high-end, health foods juggernaut now also has stores in Canada and the UK: www.wholefoodsmarket.com

Wrap your leftovers in Abeego – a handy natural cling film made from hemp, cotton fabric, beeswax and tree resin: www.abeego.ca

In your handbag

Skin Deep at ewg: cosmetic database which scores thousands of personal care products for toxicity. www.ewg.org/skindeep

At the dentist

UK and Europe

The British Society for Mercury Free Dentistry: a comprehensive list of integrative dentists throughout the country: www.mercuryfreedentistry.org.uk

Dr Goran D. Stojanovic from the Ella Clinic, London: works closely with other doctors, physiotherapists, naturopaths and nutritionists where necessary to provide a thorough health upgrade: www.theellaclinic.com/

The Paracelsus Klinik, Switzerland: leading centre for biological dentistry and medicine. For cancer patients, it offers both local and full-body hypothermia, ozone therapy, high-dose vitamins, mistletoe, energy healing and more: www.paracelsus.ch

Australia

The Australian College of Nutritional and Environmental Medicine: offers a state-by-state directory of integrative dentists: www.acnem.com.au

USA

International Academy of Oral Medicine and Toxicology: for a dentist schooled in biological dentistry including techniques for proper removal of mercury fillings: www.iaomt.org

Dr Diane Meyer: based in Illinois, she is at the forefront of holistic dentistry and patients come to her from around the world: www.holisticdentistillinois.com/

For a dentist trained in Dr Hal Huggins' natural protocol: go to www.hugginsappliedhealing.com

Dental products

Agency for Toxic Substances and Disease Registry: www.atsdr.cdc.gov/

Living Libations: natural healthy gumdrops, ionic toothbrushes and more: www.livinglibations.com

OraMD: made from 100 per cent pure botanical oils, this liquid toothpaste, mouthwash and breath freshener is endorsed by leading biological dentists around the world: www.oramd.co.uk

OraWellness: a treasure trove of information about natural solutions to dental problems, including a free interactive meridian tooth chart and a range of organic products: www.orawellness.com

Biocomp Laboratories: they will test the compatability of various dental materials with your own immune system based on serum samples: www.shslab.com

Good-gums: for a natural toothpaste alternative containing myrrh, peppermint, baking soda, French grey sea-salt, cinnamon, tea tree leaf, cranberry, vitamin C and a bioflavanoid complex: www.good-gums.com. UK and European customers can purchase the product from www.healthy.co.uk

Thermography

UK

Medical Thermal Imaging Ltd, Liverpool: www.breast-angels.com

Wholistic Medical Centre, Harley Street, London: www.wholisticmedical.co.uk

The Chiron Clinic, Harley Street, London: www.chironclinic.com

MRIs offer another radiation-free solution for monitoring your health. For those prone to claustrophobia upright and open MRI centres are now available across Britain:

www.uprightmri.co.uk/london.html

Australia and New Zealand

Note: in January 2011, the Therapeutic Goods Administration (TGA) banned thermography devices from being sold in Australia.

www.clinicalthermography.co.nz/

USA and Canada

Dr Bruce Rind: leading holistic medical doctor in Washington; along with thermography, he also offers oxygen therapies and IV nutrients: www.drrind.com

Dr Ben Johnson: co-author of the best-selling book *The Healing Codes* he devotes much of his time to spreading the word about thermography. Based in North Georgia, he helps put patients in touch with practitioners through this website: www.thermographyunlimited.com

Dr Alexander Mostovoy: a homeopathic doctor and board-certified clinical thermographer; at his busy Toronto clinic he specialises in women's health issues and breast cancer prevention: www.drmostovoy.com

Dr Jonathan V. Wright: pioneer in the research of natural treatments and founder of the Tahoma Clinic: www.tahomaclinic.com

Dr Simon Yu: weaves conventional medicine with alternative therapies at his centre in St Louis: www.preventionandhealing.com

On the phone

There are now numerous products on the market to help shield you from electromagnetic radiation, including Green 8 EMF Radiation Protection Products. Available from online retailers including www.healthy-house.co.uk and www.bioprotectivesystems.com

Beauty services

UK

Hair Organics: specialises in organic hair colours derived from natural ingredients; everything from the tea and coffee to the hand wash and cleaning products is natural and organic: www.hairorganics.co.uk

Australia

The following clinics and lifestyle retreats offer a range of natural treatments:

Gwinganna, QLD: www.gwinganna.com

Mullum Sari, NSW: www.mullumsari.com

Gaia Retreat and Spa, NSW: www.gaiaretreat.com.au

The Golden Door, NSW and QLD: www.goldendoor.com.au

Centro Health, WA: www.centrohealth.com.au

Worldwide

Neal's Yard Remedies: offers a range of holistic therapies including acupuncture, aromatherapy massage and counselling, along with high-quality essential oils, herbal remedies and organic beauty products. You'll fine branches globally: www.nealsyardremedies.com

The Organic Pharmacy: services include organic fake tan, green coffee body treatments, natural-polish pedicures and more. The Organic Pharmacy also sells a wide range of beauty products and fragrances and expert advice is on hand from their in-house homeopathic pharmacists: www.theorganicpharmacy.com

Beauty products

In the last decade there has been an explosion of natural beauty and hair-care ranges. Some of my personal favourites include Butter London (nails), Dr. Hauschka (cosmetics), Antipodes (skin care), Neal's Yard (body care), Seven Wonders Natural Hair Care and the perennial favourite, Neways.

Eco-Tan: a certified organic tan available in Australia containing no synthetic food colouring, GMO ingredients or petrochemicals: www.ecotan.com.au

Campaign for Safe Cosmetics: You can also stay abreast of the latest news by visiting: www.safecosmetics.org

Carosun: developed by Russian cosmonauts, these carnosine-rich supplements are said to offer protection from the damaging effects of cosmic radiation: www.sheridixon.com

Natracare: a brand of non-toxic feminine care products: www.natracare.com

Products to aid detoxification

For live wheatgrass

Evolution Organics: packed in individual shots and guaranteed frozen until late evening on the day of delivery. The company also sells immune-boosting supplements, enema kits and super greens for pets: www.evolutionorganics.co.uk. UK customers can purchase up to three months' worth of organic frozen wheatgrass shots.

In Perth, mum buys a fresh tray from Paul at the Mt Claremont markets on Saturdays. Australian readers can find their local market at: www.farmersmarkets.org.au

Modified Citrus Pectin: they ship worldwide: www.econugenics.com

Zeolite: Zeo Gold from Longevity Plus www.longevityplus.com and Advanced Cellular Zeolite: www.resultsrna.eu

Books

Euler, L., *Breast Cancer Cover-Up* (Online Publishing & Marketing, LLC, 2011)

Fife, B., *Oil Pulling Therapy: Detoxifying and Healing the Body Through Oral Cleansing* (Piccadilly Books, 2008)

Gittleman, A. L., *Zapped: Why Your Cell Phone Shouldn't Be Your Alarm Clock and 1,268 Ways to Outsmart the Hazards of Electronic Pollution* (HarperOne, 2011)

Gordon, G., *Detox with Oral Chelation: Protecting yourself from Lead, Mercury, and Other Environmental Toxins* (Smart Publications, 2007)

Gorman, C., *Less Toxic Alternatives* (Optimum Publishing, 2004)

Grace, J. L., *Look Great Naturally ... Without Ditching the Lipstick* (Hay House, 2012)

Hyman, M., *The Blood Sugar Solution* (Hodder & Stoughton, 2012)

Loraine, T., *Toxic Airlines* (DFT Enterprises Ltd, 2007)

Malkan, S., *Not Just a Pretty Face: The Ugly Side of the Beauty Industry* (New Society Publishers, 2007)

Meyer, D., *Pick Your Poisons 1* (RealityIsBooks, 2009)

Stacey, S. and Fairley, J., *The Green Beauty Bible: The Ultimate Guide to Being Naturally Gorgeous* (Kyle Cathie, 2008)

Somers, S., *Knockout!* (Three Rivers Press, 2010)

Woollams, C., *Oestrogen: the Killer in Our Midst* (Health Issues Ltd, 2006)

Chapter 7: Infrared Saunas and Hyperthermia

FIR saunas

Sunlighten: for an extensive range of clinically tested saunas: www.sunlighten.com

Sahara Valley: specialises in saunas with ultra-low EMR emissions: www.saharavalley.co.uk

Hyperthermia

UK and Europe

Dr Siegfried Trefzer: www.hightreemedical.com

Dr Herzog's Special Hospital: in addition to conventional cancer therapy, hyperthermia TCM, nutritional therapy, detoxification and more are on offer: www.fachklinikdrherzog.de/

Klinik St Georg: for hyperthermia, immunotherapy, homeopathy and chemotherapy: www.klinik-st-georg.de/en/

Humlegaarden: this innovative clinic north of Copenhagen offers hyperthermia, mistletoe, anthroposophical and homeopathic remedies, magnet field therapy, ozone treatment, vitamins and minerals and, in some cases, chemotherapy: www.humlegaarden.com

Australia

National Institute of Integrative Medicine (NIIM): currently studying the effects of hyperthermia when used in conjunction with chemotherapy and radiation. To be eligible for the treatment patients must become part of the Hyperthermia Clinical Research Study: www.niim.com.au/

Malaysia

Integrative Cancer Healing: with a focus on hyperthermia, this new clinic also offers vitamin C infusions, glutathione, dendritic cells, thymus, iscador, one-on-one yoga and meditation, alongside conventional cancer therapies: www.integrativecancerhealing.com

Canada

Integrated Health Clinic: offers hyperthermia along with mistletoe, acupuncture, IV minerals and more: www.integratedhealthclinic.com

DVDs and books

CANCER is Curable NOW: this feature-length documentary is packed with honest, life-affirming information about cutting-edge treatments including information about ozone, hyperthermia and intravenous vitamin C.

Kundalini Yoga: Healthy Body Fearless Spirit: renowned yoga teacher Gurmukh's spiritual workout.

Alba, J., *The Honest Life: Living Naturally and True to You* (Rodale Books, 2013)

Bollinger, T., *Cancer: Step Outside The Box* (Infinity 510^2 Partners, 2010)

Scholberg, A., *German Cancer Breakthrough: A Guide to Top German Alternative Clinics* (Online Publishing & Marketing, 2008)

Myss, C., *Why People Don't Heal and How They Can* (Bantam, 1998)

Chapter 8: There's Something About Dairy

For an extensive range of non-dairy butters, chocolates, yoghurts and nut milk bags see: www.planetorganic.com and www.wholefoodsmarket.com

For non-dairy probiotics go to www.Bodyecology.com. The website from leading digestive health specialist Donna Gates sells kefir starts, CocoBiotics and other high-quality supplements. UK residents can purchase a selection of Donna Gates's products from www.red23.co.uk

Haelan

Visit www.haelan951.com/

European customers can order Haelan 951 from Florencio Coelho in Portugal: haelan951.portugal@gmail.com

A concentrated and encapsulated form of Haelan is available for travel – Immun Plus: www.immun-plus.com

Books

Corrett, N. and Edgson, V., *Honestly Healthy* (Jacqui Small, 2012)

Daniel, K. T., *The Whole Soy Story: The Dark Side of America's Favorite Health Food* (New Trends Publishing, 2009)

Gates, D. and Schatz, L., *The Body Ecology Diet: Recovering Your Health and Rebuilding Your Immunity* (Hay House, 2011)

Plant, J., *Your Life in Your Hands* (Virgin Books, 2007)

Chapter 9: Getting in the O-zone

Practitioners

UK

Dr Thomas Marshall-Manifold: this Wimbledon-based practitioner uses ozone to treat a wide variety of viruses, infections and chronic illness: www.wimbledonclinic.co.uk

Australia and New Zealand

The Australian College of Nutritional and Environmental Medicine: also offers a state-by-state directory of integrative physicians: www.acnem.com.au

USA and Mexico

The American Academy of Ozonotherapy: dedicated to promoting research in ozonotherapy and educating the public and other health professionals about its many benefits: www.aaot.us

Dr Dan Cullum: treats patients using kinesiology, homeopathy, bio-energy testing and a wide range of ozone therapies: www.naturalhealthcenterok.com

Dr Francisco Contreras: at his renowned clinic in Tijuana Mexico, The Oasis of Hope, Dr Contreras and his team provide a range of alternative and integrative treatment options including ozone therapy, intravenous vitamin C and IPT: www.oasisofhope.com

Dr Robert Jay Rowen: regularly runs workshops on ozone therapy, hydrogen peroxide and ultraviolet blood irradiation and has educated doctors around the world about their benefits: www.secondopinionnewsletter.com; or for an extensive list of Dr Rowen's trainees: www.doctorrowen.com

Products

Ozone Generators: Dr Saul Pressman, a leading researcher in ozone therapy, sells a range of generators and accessories through his company, PlasmaFire. Complete instructions are enclosed with his products and Dr Pressman also provides free unlimited advice via email: www.plasmafire.com

Breathslim: simple breathing retraining device said to increase cellular oxygen: www.breathslim.com

Food-grade hydrogen peroxide

www.healthsolutionstechnology.com.au/

www.food-grade-hydrogen-peroxide.co.uk/

www.bobbyshealthyshop.co.uk

Books

Altman, N., *The Oxygen Prescription: The Miracle of Oxidative Therapies* (Healing Arts Press, 2007)

Borell, G., *The Peroxide Story?* (Borell, 1986)

Cavanaugh, M., *One-Minute Cure* (Think-Outside-the-Book Publishing, Inc, 2008)

Friedman, R. and Cross, M., *The Golden Ratio Lifestyle Diet* (Hoshin Media, 2011)

McCabe, E., *Flood Your Body With Oxygen* (Energy Publications, 2003)

Roguski, J. P., *The Truth about Food Grade Hydrogen Peroxide* (Under the Radar Publishing, 2009)

Scott-Mumby, K., *Cancer Research Secrets* (Scott-Mumby Wellness, 2010)

Chapter 10: Low-dose Chemotherapy and Life-saving Tests

Insulin Potentiation Therapy (IPT)

UK and Europe

Dr Thomas Kroiss at the Kroiss Cancer Centre in Vienna: www.dr-kroiss.at

USA and Mexico

Dr Francisco Contreras: www.oasisofhope.com

Dr Thomas Lodi: at An Oasis of Healing in Arizona, Dr Lodi offers low-dose chemotherapy alongside a range of holistic treatments: www.anoasisofhealing.com

Dr James Forsythe: the board-certified oncologist and homeopath recently received a lifetime achievement award: www.centurywellness.com

Dr Les Breitman: specialises in IPT: www.ipthealing.com

Cutting-edge diagnostics

UK

Practitioners who are able to facilitate RGCC analysis via Greece include Dr Wendy Denning in London, www.thehealthdoctors.co.uk and Dr Nicola Hembry in Bristol, www.drhembry.com

Denmark

Humlegaarden Cancer Clinic: now offers CellSearch® – testing of circulating tumour cells in the blood: www.humlegaarden.com

Germany

Biofocus Institute for Laboratory Medicine: for analysis of circulating tumour cells, chemo-resistance testing and 'alternative agent' testing: www.biofocus.de

Day Clinic for Prevention and Regeneration: for those who have had cancer in the past, Dr Ursula Jacob's clinic offers screening and ongoing monitoring for the presence of tumour cells in the blood. Detoxification treatments for heavy metals are also available: www.doc-jacob.com

MELISA test (for sensitivity to metals): www.invitalab.de

Greece

Research Genetic Cancer Centre (RGCC): for analysis of circulating tumour cells and cancer stem cells; branches all over the world: www.rgcc-genlab.com

USA

America Metabolic Laboratories: cancer profiling using a range of blood and urine markers including the PHI test and sensitive HCG test: www.Americanmetaboliclaboratories.net

Rational Therapeutics: provides a profile of a tumour's sensitivity and resistance to various drugs and combinations: www.rational-t.com

MELISA test: www.neuroscienceinc.com/MELISA

Japan

Dr Tsuneo Kobayashi: offers early detection – Tumour Marker Combination Assay (TMCA) – test and a range of cutting-edge therapies alongside conventional Western therapies: www.saihatsuyobou.com/lpen

Books

Forsythe, J., *Take Control of Your Cancer* (Ben Bella Books, 2012)

Chapter 11: Energy Medicine

Practitioners

UK

Paul Lennard: treats clients through a unique combination of deep-tissue massage, Chi Nei Tsang and energy healing: www.paullennard.co.uk

Australia:

Rebecca Yates: Yates uses healing frequencies to bring the body and soul back into alignment. The Reconnection® has been widely publicised and you can find a directory of practitioners here: www.thereconnection.com/

Tony Norgrove: a shamanic healer from Western Australia, Norgrove offers soul retrievals, clairvoyant readings, energy healing and more; he regularly sees clients in person, on Skype or phone, worldwide: www.thesacredtree.com.au

Dr Jerzy Dycynski (aka 'George'): a registered acupuncturist and qualified European cardiologist, Dr George uses Cardio-Stress Imaging technology to assess a patient's cardiovascular and overall health and stress levels before commencing treatment: www.remede.com.au

Tamara Gries: one of Perth's most expert bioenergy feedback analysis practitioners; also trained in reflexology and homeopathy: www.harmonyhealth.net.au

Dr Zenon Gruba: the conventionally trained physician from Melbourne offers chiropractic work, acupuncture, and MORA to energetically treat and aid in the diagnosis of patients: www.healthwiseinstitute.com.au

USA

Master Li: his unique form of healing has proven effective at treating a wide variety of illnesses deemed impossible to cure: www.u-energy.org

Brent Phillips: the inventor of The Formula for Miracles®, Brent Phillips combines the technical savvy of an MIT-trained engineer with experience of thousands of private healing sessions: www.formulaformiracles.net

Terry O'Connell: based in Idaho, O'Connell sees clients from over thirty countries and provides further training for fellow practitioners: www.thetatimes.com

PEMF

For the latest information about this exciting technology see www.pemfnow.com. Dr Garry Gordon's website provides hours of free lectures, webinars and downloads as well as selling a range of PEMF machines. See also www.somapulse.com

CDs, DVDs, online programs

Mashhur Anam (www.lifeharmonized.com): use Holographic Programs to create an 'abundance matrix'

Dr Darren Weissman (www.drdarrenweissman.com): reconnect with the power of infinite love and gratitude

Reverend Dr Iyanla Vanzant (www.innervisionsworldwide.com): Soul Food e-books, including the *Forgiveness Diet*

Sonia Choquette (www.soniachoquette.net): get in touch with your spirit guides and learn to trust your vibes

Dr Alex Loyd: thehealingcodes.com/the-master-key: unlock your 'second immune system' using Dr Alex Loyd's Master Key Technique

Kenji Kumara (www.earthangelsradio.com): quantum light weaving – for when you're 'stuck in your stuff'

Marc Ian Barasch: www.greenworld.org

Books

Braden, G., *The Isaiah Effect: Decoding The Lost Science Of Prayer And Prophecy* (Hay House, 2004)

Chan, L., *101 Miracles of Natural Healing* (Benefactor Pr, 1996)

Eden, D. and Dahlin, D., *The Little Book of Energy Medicine* (Piatkus, 2012)

Loyd, A. and Johnson, B., *The Healing Code* (Grand Central, 2011)

Myss, C., *The Creation of Health* (Bantam, 1999)

Shealy, N., *Energy Medicine: the Future of Health* (4th Dimension Press, 2011)

Swanson, C., *Life Force, the Scientific Basis* (Poseidia Press, 2009)

Virtue, D., *How To Hear Your Angels* (Hay House, 2007)

Chapter 12: Inspiring Stories

Dr Kelly Turner has recently set up a research database of unexpected remission cases (www.unexpectedremission.org) where people can go to share their story or seek inspiration. And look out for her new book, below.

Black salve: for more information about black salve see the documentary One Answer to Cancer: www.oneanswertocancermovie. com; you can also go to www.blacksalveinfo.com

Books

Richards, J., *The Topic of Cancer* (Jessica Richards, 2011)

Turner, K., *Radical Remission* (HarperCollins, forthcoming)

Chapter 13: Defeating Cancer on the Cheap

Practitioners

Dr Moshe Frankel: founder and director of Integrative Oncology Consultants; offers one-on-one appointments where patients can discuss integrative cancer solutions: www.moshefrenkelmd.com

Val Allen: uses a combination of naturopathy, homeopathy, iridology and nutrition to bring her clients back in balance: www.pnmc.com.au

Products

The Cannacig: vapour inhaler, for concentrates and oils: www.thecannacig.com/

High-quality hemp: Dixie Botanicals, based in Colorado, sells a number of high-quality cannabis-infused bath salts, oils and edibles: www.dixiebotanicals.com

Aluminium-free bicarbonate of soda: Bob's Red Mill, www.bobsredmill.com and Arm and Hammer, www.armandhammer.com

pH strips: www.bobbyshealthyshop.co.uk (also sells a variety of alkalising products including apple cider vinegar, Bob's Red Mill bicarb, chlorella and more)

Curcumin: the product Curamin contains a special form of curcumin called BCM-95®: www.curamin.com. For the latest research on curcumin and cancer see www.curcuminresearch.org

Mistletoe: the UK charity Yes to Life includes a database of practitioners who offer this treatment: www.yestolife.org.uk. Doctors in the United States and Australia can order Oral/liquid mistletoe for their patients by contacting Weleda AG: www.usa.weleda.com

Salvestrols: 1880 Life distributes high-quality salvestrols to practitioners across the UK and Ireland: www.practitionerchoice.co.uk/

Books

Carl Simonton, O., *Getting Well Again* (Bantam USA, 1980)

Collins, D., *The Top 10 Natural Cancer Cures* (Think-Outside-the-Book Publishing, LLC, 2011)

Gawler, I., *You Can Conquer Cancer* (Michelle Anderson Publishing, 2012)

Holford, P., *Say No To Cancer* (Piatkus, 2010)

Sircus, M., *Medical Marijuana* (IMVA, 2012)

Sircus, M., *Treatment Essentials* (IMVA, 2013)

Sircus, M., *Sodium Bicarbonate – Rich Man's Poor Man's Cancer Treatment.*

For the Latest Cutting-edge News

Cancer Defeated!: www.cancerdefeated.com/

The Douglass Report: www.douglassreport.com/

Green Med Info: www.greenmedinfo.com/

Health Sciences Institute: www.hsionline.com/

My website!: www.laura-bond.com

Natural News: www.naturalnews.com/

Second Opinion: www.secondopinionnewsletter.com

Underground Health Reporter:
www.UndergroundHealthReporter.com

Support Organisations

CANCERactive: the UK's number-one complementary cancer charity provides a wealth of up-to-date information on alternative and complementary treatments. It aims to arm patients and loved ones with all the available research on the causes of cancer and possible treatments and prides itself on having no vested interests: www.canceractive.com

Cancer Support WA: dance workshops, visits to Buddhist monasteries and qigong classes are just some of the activities organised by this forward-thinking charity: www.cancersupportwa.org.au

Yes to Life: UK-based charity dedicated to providing information and support for those looking for an integrative approach to cancer treatment. Yes to Life offers a dedicated support line, wellbeing workshops and online directory of practitioners trained in complementary therapies all over the world: www.yestolife.org.uk

Index